# THE BEAUTY OF
# YOGA

## Jacine Harrington

2001
Llewellyn Publications
St. Paul, Minnesota 55164-0383

FIRST EDITION
First printing, 2001

Chakra illustrations: Merle Insinga
Cover and interior model: Jacine Harrington
Cover design: Zulma Dávila
Editing and book design: Christine Snow
Photography: John Jacobs/Bear Studios

**Library of Congress Cataloging-in-Publication Data**
Harrington, Jacine.
     The beauty of yoga / Jacine Harrington. — 1st ed.
       p. cm.
     Includes bibliographical references and index.
     ISBN 0-7387-0005-3
     1. Yoga, Hatha. 2. Chakras. 3. Yoga. I. Title

RA781.7.H374 2001
613.7'046—dc21                                 2001029652

Llewellyn Worldwide does not participate in, endorse, or have any authority or responsibility concerning private business transactions between our authors and the public.

All mail addressed to the author is forwarded but the publisher cannot, unless specifically instructed by the author, give out an address or phone number.

Any Internet references contained in this work are current at publication time, but the publisher cannot guarantee that a specific location will continue to be maintained. Please refer to the publisher's website for links to author websites and other sources.

The practices, movements, and methods described in this book should not be used as an alternative to professional medical diagnosis or treatment. The author and publisher of this book are not responsible in any manner whatsoever for any injury or negative effects which may occur through following the instructions and advice contained herein. It is recommended that before beginning any treatment or exercise program, you consult your medical professional to determine whether you should undertake this course of practice.

Llewellyn Publications
A Division of Llewellyn Worldwide, Ltd.
P.O. Box 64383, Dept. 0-7387-0005-3
St. Paul, MN 55164-0383
www.llewellyn.com

Printed in the United States of America

## Acknowledgments

To my parents, who have always supported their children in all their endeavors. My special thanks for their time in editing my first drafts, and their great concern that my grammar was presentable. Their positive outlook on life serves as a role model for all to follow.

To my twin sister Katrine, with whom I share a soul-level understanding, and to my sister Sharie; the two people I know I can always count on.

To my grandmother Mary, who was a writer, painter, and a very creative person. For me, Mary emanated a love of life, and from this I learned I could be whoever I wanted to be and could do whatever I wanted to do.

To my special friends, who each offered their own unique support, always listening to my concerns, offering their own gentle wisdom. Especially to those who willingly took the time out of their busy schedules to read and comment on my first drafts of the book, asking me for more or to expand on a thought. Through your faith, the hesitations I sometimes felt were dissolved.

With grateful acknowledgement to Fazia Khan and Dr. Fedor Zelina and the respect they bring to their life partnership. Fazia, my gifted yoga instructor and spiritual advisor, helped awaken my spiritualism and continues to offer her guidance and special gift of knowledge without hesitation. Fedor, my chiropractor/naturopath, helped me through the recovery of my whiplash and with whom I took some of my first steps toward my inner journey. Without the knowledge and gentle encouragement of both these special beings, this book would not have been possible.

To my editor, Christine Snow, for including me in so many of the final decisions, always asking for and respecting my ideas on how I envisioned the book to be. This allowed me my own process of recognizing more lessons—the process of expressing my thoughts freely and openly, and then releasing the outcome. Through your efforts I trust this book will be the best it can be. Thank you.

To my photographer, John Jacobs, for your enthusiasm and professionalism in this project, and especially for your desire for perfection. Thanks for your patience and encouragement when my body wouldn't cooperate with what I wanted the camera to capture!

To my spirit guide, whom I know was always there, gently pushing me forward and giving me the determination to continue writing and the courage to open my heart and express my thoughts. At times, I felt as if knowledge was being channeled through me and it was at these times I felt your presence the most.

## Dedication

To my husband, whose quiet support serves to strengthen me.

To my children, whose unconditional faith and pride helps me realize that an open heart conquers all fear, and that we are never too old to learn and grow and to accomplish those things we want to in this life. All we need to do is try.

To my students, my source of constant inspiration, and to whom I dedicate this book. Without you, the spark that created those first thoughts leading to the beginning of this project and ending in this book would not have been ignited.

# Contents

# Part 3
# Learning the Chakras

# On a Personal Note

Physical fitness has always been a part of my life and was always something I turned to as an emotional release. As an adolescent I became interested in long-distance running as I challenged my body to exert itself at higher levels. A large part of my attraction to running was its meditative qualities—the calming process of quiet, deep-thought, long-distance running allows for. I enjoyed not only a physical "high" from the exercise, but an emotional release as well. Soon, I found I enjoyed the stretching program I developed even more, which I would do after long runs, once my muscles were warmed up and flexible. I loved the feeling of completely letting myself go into a stretch. It wasn't until years later that I realized what I was doing was an uneducated form of yoga; my body innately performing the stretches it needed.

I have always considered myself to be a student, always respecting the need to study and learn. I remember being drawn to a book when I was younger titled *The Road Less Traveled* by M. Scott Peck, M.D. The opening sentence to the book is "Life is difficult." That statement has always stuck in my mind; it captured my interest. Reading that book opened the door to my spiritual growth.

The fact that life challenges us is something I have always known. I believe we are challenged in life so that we can make mistakes, learn from our mistakes, and grow. Although I had a happy childhood, I experienced events in my young life that were difficult, including death and the inevitable learning process we go through with this experience.

I now see how these events molded me into the person I am today. It is perhaps because of these events that I seem to always be in search of myself: "Who am I?" "Why am I here?"

Through this process I have learned that difficulty does not mean that life has to be a struggle, but rather, that there is something needed to be learned. When I am put in a difficult situation, I recognize there is something I need to learn about myself at this time. I have learned to acknowledge challenges and difficulties as opportunities for growth. Knowing this makes them easier to handle. As Dr. Peck explained in his book, "Once you accept difficulty, it no longer matters." When I embrace my challenges, I know I am learning. Understanding this is the first step in knowing what it is in my past that needs releasing so that I may move forward.

The third aspect of my life that has always been a real part of who I am, even as a child, is believing in the existence of the spiritual realm— of angel guides, spirit guides, the ability to sense another realm of existence. I have experienced too many of these mystic occurrences in my life to ignore them and to not accept them as real. I have never been frightened by these events but rather simply accept them as real, and, perhaps, have taken this ability for granted. I believe that events in our lives are sometimes arranged to "shake" us up when we are not listening or paying close enough attention to what is happening around us. There is something we are not learning that we need to learn. We are ignoring information being sent to us or taking too long to move ahead on our path to learn what it is we need to learn at this stage in our lives. Such an occurrence happened to my family when we were involved in a serious car accident one sunny Sunday afternoon in July. A car traveling in the opposite direction turned directly into our path, causing a head-on collision. The reason why the car made the fatal turn into our vehicle was never established because both the driver and passenger were killed. Natural causes were ruled out after an autopsy was performed on the driver. Oddly enough, my family escaped injury, except for myself who suffered whiplash. The severity of the accident should have left us seriously injured.

Obviously, the accident was a terrifying experience for us. The whiplash aside, this event was a wake-up call for me. After two years of rehabilitation, I still suffered from pain in my neck and a nagging "knot" in my upper back, just under my right shoulder blade. I began taking a yoga class and felt immediate relief, although by evening the stiffness would return. However, one day, about two weeks into doing a regular program of yoga postures, I realized my pain was gone! There was something more to this yoga than I realized and during the time it took me to (completely) recover from my injury, my spiritual enfoldment quickened tenfold, taking me to where I am today in just a short five years. I met people who helped open doors for me, that once opened, I knew I could never turn back.

I met a special person, Kathy Roseborough, who invited me to one of her meditation groups. A clairvoyant and spiritual healer, Kathy was instrumental in helping me take my first steps into inner work and healing, discovering inner truths by literally peeling away protective layers I had placed around myself throughout the years. I was then introduced to two people who played the most significant roles in my spiritual growth, Dr. Fedor Zelina and Fazia Khan. Fedor became my chiropractor/naturopath and Fazia introduced me to her approach to yoga. Within weeks of practicing the postures Fazia taught me, my pain and muscle tenderness caused by the whiplash was gone. What also attracted me to this form of yoga was the fact that I was introduced to a method of working with my chakras alongside working with my physical body. I was familiar with working with my chakras, and Fazia's approach was refreshing. After years of enjoying fitness of various sorts, for the first time I enjoyed a complete and "whole" body experience. There was something very intriguing to this yoga and I knew a wanted more!

Studying yoga was a natural step for me. I approached Fazia to formally teach me the art of what I like to call chakra yoga. With my study I discovered yoga's gentleness and beauty. I discovered the strength of yoga and how I was becoming stronger physically, emotionally, and mentally. I allowed my inner self to open up and walk on a path of self-discovery. Fazia is a part of this book and I acknowledge with gratitude that the knowledge I gained from Fazia's teachings and her continual, gentle support has helped in the creation of this book. Chakra yoga helped me go beyond the events happening in my life to understanding them and how they created the person I have become. There have been many other people I have met on this journey, who each in their own unique way have helped me along my path. I recognize these meetings were not merely chance but incidents that were meant to happen.

We all have our lessons to learn and we are here on earth to learn them. It is easier for us to learn our lessons on the "earth plane" or "earth school," because it is on earth that we interact with others. It is through interaction that we learn about ourselves and how we react to situations. When my buttons are pushed, I know there are issues of my own that need to be dealt with. Instead of being angry with people who upset me, I try to thank them. This isn't always easy, but I do believe we are here to help each other and that sometimes others are used as instruments to bring forward issues we need to learn. We have the choice to decide how to deal with our issues.

I do not allow myself to get "pulled in" to other people's issues or their negativity, nor do I let negative emotions "settle" into my being. Learning to live from a place of peace within is the essence of true health. "Life" happens that can interrupt this sense of calm, so we must learn to release on all levels in order to clear and balance. Chakra yoga allows me to do this. I live my life being aware of how I choose to interact with people and how I choose to live. I recognize that my fears are my weaknesses, and that these weaknesses are what I need to work on. I am sometimes afraid, but I still try to take a step forward into the unknown, to see how it feels, and with it take my steps toward growth. I know this is an opportunity and that fear is necessary only as a signal to stop and listen to what is happening around me; to pause and pay attention, that something needs more work.

When things seem to happen in my life over and over again, I know it is a lesson I have not yet learned. You will be tested to see if you have learned your lesson. New situations will be arranged to bring the issues back into your life. When you are tested, take this as your opportunity to stand in your power and be strong.

One lesson I have learned is to let go of worry. I have changed that pattern in my life. There was a time that worry visited me often, and when it did, I began to worry needlessly over things I had no control over. The more I worried, the more habit-forming it became. I now try to live in, and come from, "the moment." I listen to and follow my instincts. The more I do this, along with trust and acknowledgement, my instincts become sharper. Things happen for a reason over which we usually have little power. Keep yourself open so that you are shown that reason. Answers will come, and when they do, acknowledge them with gratitude. When you become aware of this process, you develop the insight to break away from the damaging effects worry can have on your body.

Writing a book was not something I ever imagined myself doing. My search for inner truth began many years ago and with this search came the desire and need to write down my experiences, thoughts, and dreams. When I began studying yoga, my spiritual enfoldment was put into fast forward and logging my experiences became essential as a part of my learning experience. Throughout my teaching, my personal diaries have become a part of the knowledge I share in my classes, while I continue to learn and continue to keep a diary of my thoughts and experiences. Soon, I could feel the beginnings of a book emerging, and this excited me. It was not until my students began requesting me to write a book, produce a video, or record tape cassettes for them so that they could practice their yoga at home on their own that the idea to write a book became a reality. I felt that a message was being sent to me and that I needed to listen! When I did, the desire to express and share my knowledge became very strong and something I could not ignore. I was once told by someone, whom I consider to be a very enlightened being, that "the decisions I make in this life will affect me for thousands of lives to follow." His advice to me was to make my decision wisely. I feel this in my life, and that the decision to write this book is a positive one that can help many people.

There are some things I follow as basic truths in my life:

- Be your own person. Have the confidence to be who you want to be and to do what you want to do. You have no one to impress but yourself.

- Your thoughts count, so be careful what you think or ask for. You are sending a message out to the universe, and you will be answered.

- Don't get drawn into any form of negativity and try not to worry. These things only serve to steer you off course and impede your growth.

- Release your past by forgiving others. Forgiveness leads the way to love and love has the power to conquer ill feelings. You may not agree with the decisions of others, but you can support them. Remember we are all on our own path of self-discovery and our rates of growth are different.

- And last of all, follow your instincts. Try to live your life with an open heart and listen to it whenever you can. This is where your answers come from.

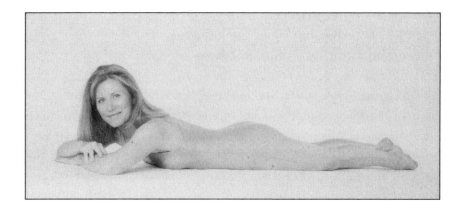

# Introduction

Anyone who has attended even one yoga class knows that yoga is much more than just another method of physical fitness. Yoga reduces stress and tension in your body and, through regular practice, helps the body become strong and supple. In this book, I take you one level deeper and invite you to explore your emotions and feelings as you perform physical postures, helping you discover how you are physically connected to those emotions and feelings. This is done through "chakra" work, a method of exploring and becoming in tune with your inner thoughts and feelings—your emotional body.

Chakras are energy centers that store your emotions, feelings, and thoughts, both positive and negative. Often, we are unaware that we hold on to negative emotions, especially when they are small or seemingly insignificant. This can be dangerous. Holding on to even the most minor negative emotions can lead to a build-up of negative energy. Unaware of this build-up within ourselves, these emotions can become trapped in our bodies, blocking the path to true inner peace and happiness. Keeping these emotions trapped in our body traps us into our past; we are not able to move forward. Opening and balancing your chakras helps you to recognize or become aware of negative energy and/or issues that have become trapped and that no longer serve your purpose. Revealing this energy to yourself and acknowledging it as real is the first step in helping you to release.

Chakra work gives you the tools needed to take charge and release this energy, promoting inner healing and better all-around health, allowing you to move forward in life. I refer to this approach to yoga as chakra yoga. I believe that as you release on a physical level through postures, you also release on an emotional level. I base my yoga classes on this premise and help my students to recognize this happening in their bodies, so that they can gain more benefit from their practice of yoga. Chakra yoga has become a way of life for me, and through it my path of self-discovery is less obstructed and my rate of growth accelerated.

Although I wrote this book largely to demonstrate the postures and what you can learn from them, I want to convey a very important message concerning my philosophy to chakra yoga. My belief is that our mind, emotions, and physical well-being are connected. The idea to practice the discipline of yoga often intimidates people, because it is surrounded by many misunderstandings. This book is my attempt to bridge the gap, erase the misunderstanding, to help you discover yoga's beauty and gentleness. With all the benefits yoga has to offer, discover how strong your body can become, both physically and emotionally. Go one step further and begin to feel yourself become reconnected to your spirit—to your "self" and "who" you are. Yoga is not a mystical practice whereby you are required to be incredibly flexible in order to participate. You do not need to be able to "do" or "be" anything but yourself and simply have the desire to lead a healthier, stronger, more fulfilling life.

I talk to too many people who do not understand why they are always sick or feeling unhealthy even though they spend an enormous amount of time, effort, and money on their physical well-being through nutrition and exercise. While this is all essential to our health, I have learned there is one important step missing. That is, if we do not attend to our emotional and mental well-being, our physical body cannot heal itself completely.

This book is especially for those who seem to always have a lot of stress in their lives and do not know how to let go. Chakra yoga can teach you how to learn from your stress as you find out where it comes from. It is not until then that you can begin to release the negative energy from your life. This is what it means to "discover" yourself. For me, knowing who I am comes from understanding where I came from—my weaknesses and my fears.

Chakra work is about self-discovery and chakra yoga can help speed up your journey of self-discovery. I practice this form of yoga because I feel nourished and strengthened on all levels. I am left feeling wonderfully energized and invigorated as I open up and prepare myself to face challenges emotionally, physically, and mentally. I allow myself to bring forth and release inner fears within an environment I feel completely safe and comfortable in. I deal with only those issues I feel I comfortably can at the time. This book is my way to share this information with you, helping you discover who you are as you begin your own journey. For those of you already on your way, I hope to provide you with a method of tuning into your body on a deeper level, helping you to reach your emotional, mental, and physical potential.

I believe that to gain the most benefit from yoga you need to come face to face with your weaknesses, which are almost always your life lessons, as you discover the root to those weaknesses. You learn life lessons and how to overcome fears in order to grow and continue on your path. To stay focused on your needs, you learn to go inward. From here situations that would normally cause you stress no longer upset you or throw you off balance. Going inward to deal with life's stresses allows you to draw from a calm and centeredness created within, instead of using external sources, which can often be distorted and vague.

It is important for you to have an understanding of the chakras in order for you to work with them along with your postures. For this reason the book is written in three parts. Part 1, "Preparing for Yoga," discusses everything you need to know to begin a yoga program. Part 2, "Practicing Your Yoga," demonstrates and instructs you on how to do the breathing exercises, limbering and spine-stretching postures, counter postures, and postures for each of the chakras. Part 3, "Learning the Chakras," outlines each of the seven chakras and what they mean.

I suggest you read the book in its entirety before beginning a yoga program. Then go back to the postures, referring to the section on "Learning the Chakras" as needed. My hope is that you use this book in a way that is most useful to you. There need not be a lot of structure to your yoga program. Look past the structure so you may discover the gentleness of yoga and bring it within.

I begin this book on a personal note, with why I needed to write it and what I have learned through yoga and chakra balancing. My practice of yoga has brought me to where I am today, as I continue to look down my road of self-discovery with anticipation and open arms.

I have thoroughly enjoyed the experience of writing this book. Once started, I couldn't seem to turn off the flow of information that kept coming. At times the information felt like it was being channeled through me. I often received inspiration through interaction with friends, family, my students, and even strangers.

Understanding that events happen for a reason and that people come into our lives to help teach us something is a premise I have always lived my life by. I hadn't realized the importance this role played in the creation of this book, however, until I happened to read *The Celestine Vision* by James Redfield, given to me by a friend of mine. Conversations and information often seemed to arrive at just the right time to complete a train of thought or a chapter in the book, or would spark a new thought or idea that seemed to complement the information already included in a particular chapter. Perhaps, too, this book arrived at just the right time to help make this concept clearer to me. As I recognize these coincidences, I know I am growing and learning as I write, and that this is a part of my own self-discovery. I acknowledge this with gratitude.

It is my sincere wish that you find joy and a clearer understanding of who you are through chakra yoga as I have. Keep an open heart. Know my thoughts are with you as you take your steps toward living life more fully.

# Part 1
# PREPARING
# FOR YOGA

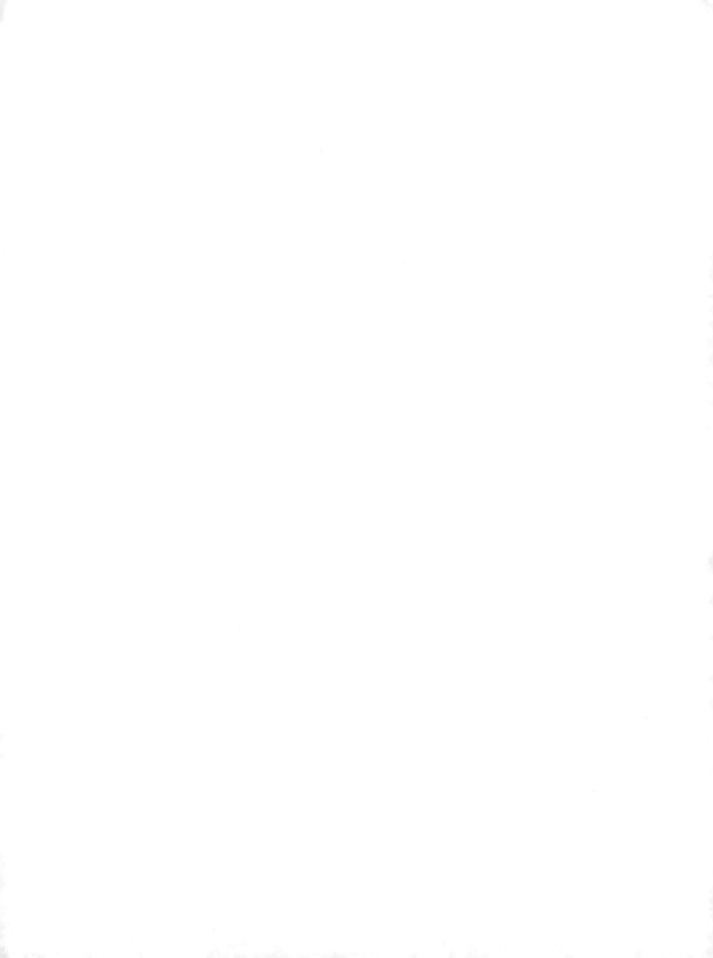

Chapter 1

# Getting Ready to Begin

Often, the hardest part in committing yourself to an exercise program is getting started. With yoga you will find a difference. Once your body has experienced the exhilarating effects yoga has to offer, you won't want to stop. Beginning a yoga program is easier than you think. All you need is a quiet spot, a comfortable blanket, some soothing music, and you are ready to go. Take the time to experience yoga's benefits and its gentleness, beauty, and grace.

## When Should I Do Yoga?

If you choose to do your program in the morning, take a bath first to warm your muscles, making them less tense. Your physical progress may be a little slower if postures are done in the morning since your muscles are less flexible at this time of day. However, the benefit of doing postures now is that you will feel great the rest of the day and be more willing to continue your program each morning.

Doing yoga in the evening is equally as beneficial. The muscles are not as stiff, allowing you to go further into your postures. You will get a restful sleep and you will wake up feeling refreshed. It is best to do your yoga after a light meal, or if possible, an hour or so after eating. It may be uncomfortable to do postures on a full stomach.

Ideally, yoga should be practiced daily, however, with our busy lifestyles this is often not possible. You will find a schedule that suits you best. You will notice how yoga allows you to honor your needs, while allowing you to balance them with the demands of a busy life. In yoga, you learn to take the time to listen to yourself—to tune in. You are taught to listen to the needs of your body. If you only have time for a few exercises some days, do the ones you feel do you the most good. Always listen to your body to see what postures it needs that day. Remember, yoga is not about being hard on yourself or judging yourself for not having time to exercise. (My own schedule consists of doing pranayamas, chakra work, and meditation for 30 minutes in the morning. My postures are done later in the day as my schedule permits, usually in the early evening once my family has settled in after dinner.)

## Where Do I Do Yoga?

All you need is a quiet place with little interruption. Wear comfortable clothing and lie on a blanket to protect your face when doing stomach postures. Avoid doing postures on a concrete floor, even if the floor is covered by carpeting. Concrete floors are cold and hard and can cause injury to your spine. If possible, lie on an exercise mat placed under your blanket for added cushioning.

## Yoga Equipment

Yoga has become a popular form of exercise in our Western society, and along with its popularity, many "Western" aids have been designed with the intention of making the experience with the postures more comfortable and pleasurable. Although not necessary, these items can help you be more comfortable and confident, allowing you to perform some postures with greater ease.

Probably the most highly marketed item is the yoga mat or sticky mat, available through many yoga studios. These mats are designed to

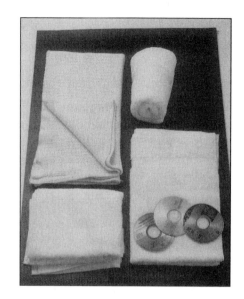

reduce slipping or sliding during the standing postures. I have used a sticky mat, and while it is great in preventing slippage, and therefore helps make the posture easier to perform, I find standing on a bare floor or carpet in my bare feet equally suffices, as do many of my students.

I personally prefer a more cushioned exercise mat and recommend using one. It is gentler on your spine and knees when doing the postures. If you do not have a mat, a blanket or towel would work as well. Place the blanket under your knees for added cushioning when needed or under your spine for others. The important thing to note is there is no right or wrong way. Follow your own instincts as to what will work best for you, listening to your body and what feels right.

Other items on the market are specific yoga aids to help you more easily get into a posture. These are such things as belts, bolsters, and specially sized towels or blankets. Again, these items are not necessarily needed but can help you be more comfortable when trying to get into certain postures, especially if you find your body can't "get" to where it is supposed to "be." (*Note:* I personally do not use these special yoga aids, other than a plain towel, and do not promote them in my classes. I inform all my students of the equipment that is available and suggest to them, especially in the beginning, not to go out and purchase all this extra "stuff" until the need arises. To date, not one of my students has purchased any of this specialized equipment.)

One needs to be careful, however, not to use these aids as a quick fix or in order to fulfill that sense of instant gratification we all tend to want or be fooled into thinking we need. My philosophy to yoga is to only go as far as is comfortable when performing any posture. You do not receive any further benefit in pushing yourself beyond this point. This teaches you patience. Your muscles have a memory and your flexibility will come back. Performing your yoga program without the use of aids allows you to stay more focused during your yoga program, almost as if in a meditation, listening to your body, only going as far as is comfortable. A good yoga instructor will watch you and let you know when to stop, allowing your muscles a chance to respond to the stretch. Slowly, over time, your muscles will become more flexible, and you will find you can go into a posture further.

There is no competition in yoga and it's okay if you can't get into the full extension of a posture. Part of learning yoga is to be able to "release" yourself into the knowledge that you don't have to be where everyone else is, and to praise yourself for where you are. As you advance slowly by simply listening to your body, deciphering when you are able to go further into a stretch, you get far more satisfaction than being able to do the posture by the use of an aid, in my experience.

There are instances when I recommend to my students the use of a towel to help them get into a posture more easily. A towel can be used in a belt fashion to help you reach areas on your body you normally could not reach. It can be used to raise a body part or used to rest a body part on during a posture, helping you perform the posture more easily. Throughout the posture chapters in the margins, I have added suggestions, where applicable, where the use of a towel may be helpful.

The point I would like to stress is that it is not necessary for you to purchase any special equipment in order to perform your yoga routine. There are aids available to help make your routine more comfortable, and it is up to you to decide what will work best for you.

## Be Gentle On Yourself

Don't rush your yoga. Go into each posture carefully, being aware of where each part of your body needs to go. Hold each posture for a few seconds as you listen to your body. This makes the posture more effective and helps to ensure that you will not experience muscle soreness or fatigue once your yoga is finished. The slow pace and gentleness of yoga gives you greater control over the positioning, safety, and efficiency of each pose.

Always maintain an awareness of protecting your body during the postures. When doing any standing postures, such as the Standing Chest Opener, or any seated postures, such as the Seated Forward Bend Series, always keep your knees slightly bent in an unlocked position to protect them. Locking your knees or overextending them causes undue strain on the knee and the muscles and tendons surrounding it. During any lying postures, such as the Locust or the Leg Raises, squeeze your buttock muscles to support your lower back. Be aware of your lower back at all times. You should never feel strain in your lower back. If you do, you are pushing yourself beyond your comfort level.

Be aware of your comfort level and hold the posture for only as long as your comfort level permits, giving you the opportunity to look within. You are able to feel how you respond to the posture both on a physical and emotional level. Holding a posture strengthens your body physically and allows for heightened body awareness. Try not to force yourself into a posture. Your body receives no benefit from pushing yourself into a stretch, causing unnecessary strain on the body. Carefully bring yourself out of the posture. Once again, be aware of where each part of your body is and where it needs to go. Jarring yourself out of a position may cause injury, especially to the lower back. You may also lose some of the benefit received from the posture. Come out of the posture gently and slowly, staying in your center.

## Remember to Breathe

Maintain an awareness of your breath throughout your yoga routine, allowing your breathing and body to move together. Do the postures properly, breathing into each stretch and breathing while holding the posture to relax your muscles. Imagine sending your breath to the muscles being stretched. Soon, you will notice these muscles relaxing, allowing you to stretch a little further, making your body more flexible.

Breathe normally throughout the postures, never forgetting to breathe. There is a tendency to hold your breath while holding a posture.

Holding your breath causes the muscles to stiffen. Instead, learn to relax while in the postures, breathing into each one. This improves the supply of oxygen to the muscles, allowing them to relax and stretch further.

Pause and rest for a few breaths between postures. Allow your body to balance and assimilate what it has learned while letting your muscles recover from the stretch. Experience the gentleness of yoga. You don't need to experience pain, fatigue, or sore muscles.

Do not be alarmed if you feel a little dizziness during the postures in the beginning. Some postures send a rush of blood to the head, such as the Shoulder Stand, or any posture where the head is lowered back, such as the Fish or the Camel. This may cause a slight headache or dizzy feeling. As well, you receive a high intake of oxygen during pranayamas, something your body may not be accustomed to and so may cause a slight headache. If the dizziness persists after a couple of weeks of doing your yoga program, consult your doctor before continuing.

Chapter 3 will discuss pranayamas in more detail and chapter 4 describes some basic relaxation and breathing exercises.

## Stay Focused

Concentrate on what you are doing, especially during the balancing postures, such as the Eagle Pose or the Tree Pose. Moving rapidly or laughing during a posture will cause you to lose concentration and move out of your center. You then will not receive as much benefit from the posture.

Lastly, resist the temptation to compare yourself to others. Your personal progress is important to you and only you. It does not matter how far you can or cannot go into a stretch. Your muscles have a memory and with practice, patience, and persistence, your ability to advance into the postures will come. Release the need to be competitive and enjoy the gentleness of the yoga. Yoga is not about being competitive with yourself or anyone else. For this reason, it is a good idea to close your eyes and stay focused, centered, and in tune to the needs of your body, never judging yourself or others.

## Beginner or Advanced

A beginner can safely do most of the postures demonstrated in the book. Remember, however, to listen to your body and go into a posture only as far as your comfort level permits. Some postures include advanced positions. Once you can do the basic posture smoothly and without strain, move into the advanced position. Allow your body to progress naturally at its own pace.

## Special Advice

### Medical Notes

**Before beginning any type of exercise program, you should always consult your physician first.** If you suffer from any sort of medical problem, it is especially important to consult your doctor before beginning a yoga program. In most cases, yoga can help your problem, however, it is up to your doctor to tell you it is okay. There are many yoga books available that deal specifically with medical ailments and those postures that will help them.

A common medical complaint I hear from my students, friends, and family is one related to lower back problems. Yoga is a wonderful release for back problems of any sort, however, once again, I must stress the importance of first consulting with a doctor before beginning a yoga program at this time. Any back problem or neck problem stemming from weak, tense, or tight muscles can be helped by yoga. Yoga postures deal with the spine and the muscles along the spine. It helps to stretch, balance, and strengthen these muscles so that they can support the spine in the manner they were intended. Yoga is an excellent preventative approach to help strengthen and stretch these muscles.

A special note with regard to back problems: If you are experiencing stiffness and spasms due to a back injury, now is NOT the time to start yoga. Allow your back the rest it needs so that it can heal naturally. Once the stiffness is gone, and your doctor gives you the okay, begin strengthening your back muscles by doing the limbering-up postures found in chapter 8.

### A Woman's Moon Cycle

In yoga, a woman's menstrual cycle is referred to as her "moon cycle." If you are on the first day of your moon cycle, you should not do any postures. It isn't necessary to exercise as vigorously at this time as there is already an energy flowing naturally in your body. If you feel the need to do yoga, do only the "opening" postures, such as the Goddess Pose or the Fish Posture, and "backward" postures, such as the Camel. These poses will keep the energy flow of your moon cycle moving in the natural direction. After the first day, it is okay to continue your yoga program, once again concentrating on the opening and backward postures. Listen to your body and its needs.

The moon cycle is the time for relaxation and meditation; to be still. Women are in their power at this time, and their intuitive energy is very high. Inner knowledge and wisdom comes through when women take the time to listen. Take some quiet time for yourself. Listen to your wisdom. Honor your body and your cycle. Major changes happen in your body at this time. A regular practice of yoga can help regulate your moon cycle to three days, which is considered to be a normal cycle range in yoga.

## Pregnancy

Relaxation and breathing exercises are useful for a pregnant woman, preparing her for childbirth. It is okay to do yoga postures during pregnancy with the exception of a few. For example, the Locust posture should never be done during pregnancy as it can lead to a miscarriage almost immediately. You should also stay away from postures where you lie on your stomach for the simple reason that they may be uncomfortable. It is important to always be aware of any discomfort in your body and of what your body is telling you. Pregnancy brings many changes to the body that can affect each woman differently. Certain postures may feel wonderful for some pregnant women but not for others.

There are many postures that are beneficial as they help strengthen the muscles in the back and the pelvis floor. Such postures as the Staff Pose, Goddess Pose, Fish, and the Camel's sitting variation are recommended. The Butterfly Pose and the squat used to enter the Elephant help to open the hips, preparing the body for childbirth. It is important to note that the muscles in the hips and pelvic floor become very relaxed in the late stages of pregnancy and can be easily strained. When doing postures during any stage of your pregnancy, take it slow and easy.

Chapter 2

# Nutrition

I am always astonished as to how little people know about the foods they eat and how important they are to their general state of health. Food is more that just something to fill you up and to enjoy. It is fuel for your body and it is what gives your body energy. The basis of your health is the diet you eat. The quality of nutrients in the foods you eat is directly related to the quality of your health. The more nutritious and wholesome your diet is, the healthier you will be.

The philosophy I follow and explain to my students is one which maintains a healthy, balanced attitude toward how you live your life, respecting your body with regard to the foods you consume. Eating wholesome, nutritious foods will help maintain a healthy body to support daily exercise as well as your busy lifestyle.

The study of yoga encompasses the whole body including a "yogic" diet to help restore peace to the body and mind. Not all authorities of yoga philosophy are in agreement over what constitutes a proper diet, however, the foundation to a yogic diet is the more natural the food is, the more *prana*, or life force, it will have, and therefore, the better it will be for your body. This is often referred to as the *satvic*, or whole and natural, diet. These are foods such as fresh vegetables and fruits, grains, legumes, whole-grain breads and pastas, cheese, milk, butter, tofu, and honey.

Following the philosophy of the satvic diet, the intake of meat, fish, or poultry is not highly stressed because the amount of prana found in these foods is considered to be lower than that found in natural foods. However, with the demands placed on our bodies by modern-day society, an active lifestyle, and particularly stress, many of us need the protein we get from meat, fish, and poultry. Protein supplies your body with energy once it has used the carbohydrate and fat cells reserved for this function. When you are active and/or under a lot of stress, your body is depleted of its energy faster than normal. If you have not supplied your body with the necessary "fuel" to sustain its energy, you will feel depleted. Milk, eggs, rice, soy products, beans, and lentils are other good sources of protein but are not as high as in a small portion of meat. The type of lifestyle you lead and the amount of stress placed on your body physically, mentally, or emotionally will determine the amount and type of protein your body needs. Protein is not stored in the body, but even so, we do not need as much as we think we do. Eating a little bit throughout your day will keep your energy level sustained and balanced. Once again, listen to your body and its needs.

Water makes up a large part of your body weight, and it is required for almost every function in the body—from digestion to temperature control to eliminating waste. Many authorities recommend drinking at least six to eight glasses of water daily. This can be difficult to do. Try keeping a glass of water or a water bottle with you and sip on it slowly throughout your day. You will be surprised at how quickly you can drink six to eight glasses of water when you are not paying attention to it. Anyone wishing to lose weight will benefit from this because water decreases the craving for snacking by giving you a sense of being full.

Whenever possible, choose organically grown foods. Try to avoid processed foods. They are considered to be "empty" of any nutritional value and will not provide you with the necessary energy your body requires to prepare it for the demands of your day.

As a mother of three young children, I often find it difficult to follow a yogic diet; my difficulty stems from finding enough foods to please my children, my husband, and myself. However, when I do eat foods that are natural and pure, I always feel better for it. Recently, I have discovered a wonderful vegetarian cookbook following the satvic principles called *The Yoga Cookbook*, created by the staff of the International Sivananda Yoga Centers. This cookbook offers a wide range of delicious, easy-to-cook meatless dishes that even the kids enjoy. I especially enjoy their suggestions for a "yogic start to the day."

Eating and living a healthy lifestyle is important to your health. The more natural the foods are that you eat and the higher the quality of their nutrients, the more you are doing to nourish your body and maintaining your general good health. Balance your lifestyle with plenty of activity and rest, work and play, good food and fun!

# Part 2

# PRACTICING
# YOUR YOGA

Chapter 3

# Pranayamas

The branch of yoga I practice and teach is hatha yoga. Hatha yoga, meaning "union through determined effort" in Sanskrit, balances and strengthens the body through physical exertion and includes the spiritual element we all come to expect from yoga. The physical element of stretching my body, along with the spiritual element, is what attracted me to hatha yoga. With a background in long-distance running and aerobics, my body craves the exhilaration of energizing itself through physical fitness. Hatha yoga provides an efficient source of physical postures to satisfy this craving, builds a healthy and strong body, uses breathing exercises to calm the emotions, and calls for mental concentration to strengthen the mind. All of these aspects make up what is known as the spiritual practice of yoga, or *Sadhana*. Sadhana includes these three areas:

- *Pranayamas*, or breathing exercises, to help quiet the emotions and the mental body.
- *Asanas*, or postures, to strengthen the physical body.
- Meditation to remove stress and to help center you and connect to your higher self.

Chakra yoga works to open, activate, and balance your chakras—energy centers that run along your spine—within these three areas of Sadhana. (Chakras are explained in detail in part 3.)

Pranayamas, or breathing exercises, provide the foundation to yoga, our breath being the most important food for our body and mind. The function of breathing draws oxygen into the body and sends it to the bloodstream. Breathing also expels waste, in the form of carbon dioxide, from your body and cleanses the blood of toxins. The cells in your body are repaired and energized as you send them oxygen. It is for this reason that pranayamas are a prime focus in yoga and why breathing is important during the postures.

*Prana* means "breath" or "life force"; *ayamas* means "pause" or "control." It is believed by many who practice yoga that with more prana, or breath, the more alert and energetic you become. You can think more clearly. Your body is more relaxed, your mind calm. You have a heightened awareness of who you are and a stronger connection between your body, mind, and emotions. You are more in tune with your inner self and your higher self. You hear your inner voices and messages more clearly.

Controlling prana, that is, how you inhale and exhale, has an effect on your emotions. With practice, your breathing pattern can control your emotions. It is important for you to realize this. For example, when you are angry, excited, or nervous, your breathing is faster and heavier. When you are calm, your breathing is more relaxed and slow. You can learn to calm your emotional body when you are in uncomfortable situations by learning to calm or slow down your breathing. This is what pranayamas teach you. Becoming familiar with the pranayamas, or breathing exercises, outlined in the next chapter give you techniques to help you learn how to you calm your mind, your emotions, and your physical body so that you can stay centered and clearly focus on the task at hand.

The many benefits of pranayamas and regulating your breathing include the following:

- Calms the mind.

- Clears the sinuses.
- Prolongs life by slowing down the heart.
- Aids in digestion and purification of the blood, which improves circulation, your complexion, and energy.
- Increases oxygen intake, which gives you a sense or feeling of satisfaction or fullness.
- Helps you be more alert and to think more clearly.
- Helps you become more aware of discomfort in your body. Adjust your body if you feel discomfort during pranayamas. You can stay centered while shifting your body when necessary.
- Helps you become aware of being more open in the chest area.
- Helps you have the experience of spirit because your mind is calm and your emotions are settled and balanced, resulting in a body/mind integration.
- Helps you reach a quiet, all-knowing place inside—your "place of center" where your answers come from. If you have a life question, ask it before you go into relaxation and pranayamas. The answer will come, tapping into your inner wisdom.
- Heals you emotionally, mentally, and physically.
- Slows down time and calms your mind so that you live "in the moment."
- Helps you become centered and not swayed by others' negative thoughts. This stays with you throughout the day. You can bring yourself into this place of centeredness at any time through your calming breath.

There are many pranayamas to choose from. All concentrate on the breath coming through the nostrils. The nostrils act as a filter, cleansing the breath of impurities. The breath is also warmed and moistened as it passes through your nostrils, making it less invasive to your body. Breathing through your nose, both inhaling and exhaling, helps start a "communication" within your body—an intercellular communication. This helps you to become aware of your breath, bringing an awareness, strengthening your connection between the mind and emotions.

It is best to close your eyes during pranayamas, helping you to remain focused within that place of calm and centeredness. This teaches you to be gentle with yourself and not to judge yourself or those around you. We are not meant to judge others or ourselves. Rather, we are meant to have peace of mind and to be honest with ourselves, while being gentle.

Begin and end your spiritual practices with some manner of relaxation, such as the Opening to Postures Visualization in chapter 5, or by using any of the breathing exercises listed in chapter 4. Pranayamas help you get centered and connected to your higher self. It is from here that you are led into meditation. When you move into meditation, you are able to observe what happens in your life. This is how you learn your lessons and how you grow. It is important to check in with yourself regularly. "Did I learn that lesson I needed to learn?" "Are my old thought-patterns and belief systems still around, not allowing me to grow?" Observe yourself honestly and with a sharp eye. Follow your inner guide so that you may move forward in your life and onto a higher path. When you receive messages or confirmation when in meditation, know this information comes to you as a result of learning to recognize yourself—loving yourself, acknowledging yourself, and sitting in appreciation of who you are.

When you have completed your pranayamas, you are ready to enter the postures while in this meditative state. Your body is now able to receive more benefit from the movements because you are now in tune with yourself and your body. You are calm and focused, and it is from this place of centeredness that you are able to find a connection to your emotional body. You are able to listen and hear the needs of your body—the body/mind integration—because pranayamas teach you to spend some time with yourself, to listen to your body, your thoughts, feelings, dreams, and aspirations. You begin to recognize your spirit—that sense of "who" you are. When you do not take the time for relaxation and pranayamas in the beginning of your program, you will only receive the physical benefits, without the effects of the inner work that happens on a deeper level.

Always try to allow at least 10 minutes at the end of your program for relaxation by doing the Closing Meditation in chapter 5. Remember, you release on an emotional level as well as on a physical one, even though you may not be aware of such a release. Relaxing the body and mind after yoga allows this information to come forward. Relaxation helps create a space for healing, gives you that quiet moment needed to acknowledge your growth, and allows new knowledge to feel comfortable in your body. With your breath, old thought-forms leave the body, creating space for the new.

Chapter 4

# Relaxation and Breathing Exercises

## Connected Breath

The Connected Breath is a nice way to begin your relaxation as it quickly draws your awareness inward as you focus on your breath. The simple act of focusing on your breath allows the body to relax. As you breathe slowly, connect your inhaling breath to your outgoing breath so it becomes one fluid motion. Stay focused on your breath and follow it all the way. Feel yourself begin to let go, releasing any stress in your body. The Connected Breath can help you learn to listen and trust your inner guidance and intelligence.

**Figure 4-1**

*Sit up as straight as you can to allow for an energy flow through your body. As you breathe in and out, breathe slowly and completely.*

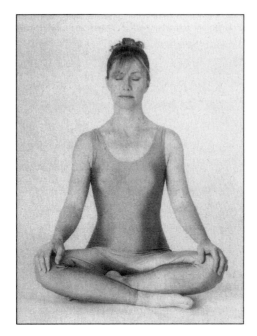

1. Come into a comfortable sitting or lying position, whichever is most comfortable for you, and begin breathing through your nostrils. Your spine should be straight to allow for energy flow through your body.

2. Close your eyes. Allow your body to relax. Consciously relax your entire body—your physical, mental, and emotional body. Continue breathing through your nostrils, filling your lungs completely. Feel your lungs expanding and filling with oxygen. You begin to feel your body relaxing. (See Figure 4-1.)

3. When you exhale, completely empty the air from your lungs. You are breathing calmly and slowly. This is not an exaggerated breath. Take about 20 of these slow, connected breaths into your lungs.

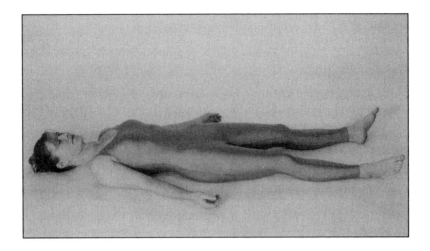

**Figure 4-2**

*As you continue to breathe slowly and completely, start to focus your energy on your physical body, relaxing your entire body.*

## Relaxation Posture (*Savasana*)

Feel yourself letting go in the Relaxation Posture as your body becomes completely still. Focus primarily on your physical body, letting go of any stress in your body. As you breathe through your nostrils, look to your breath and follow it all the way. Allow your body to come into a state of complete relaxation.

1. Lie on the floor with your feet shoulder width apart. Your arms are at your side, about 2–3 inches away from your body. The palms of your hands should face up in a receiving position. (See Figure 4-2.)

2. Walk your shoulders down from your ears with the intention to relax—and you do. Consciously relax your neck and shoulders. Start to focus your energy, allowing the focus to be primarily on your physical body, relaxing your entire physical body.

3. Continue lying completely still for 10 breaths.

## Body Parts Relaxation (*Savasana II*)

This is designed to help relax your entire body. You may feel a warm, tingling sensation in the parts you have started to relax as energy flows there—the energy you are sending to your body. When you focus your attention somewhere on the body, you send your energy there. Be aware that where you place your attention, your energy, you also place your love; loving yourself and that part of your body. You begin to feel the energy awakening in your body. Your body is becoming more and more relaxed. You begin to feel tension and tightness leave your body. Allow yourself to be in the stillness of your own being and to lie in silence.

1. Continue to lie in the Relaxation Posture (see Figure 4-2, page 23) and breathe through your nostrils. As you slowly go through the various body parts, consciously relax them as they are mentioned.

2. Focus your attention to the bottom of your feet and consciously relax your feet. Move your attention up to your ankles and relax your ankles. Move up to your calves and knees, relaxing your calves and knees. Move up to your thighs, relaxing your thighs.

3. Continue breathing through your nostrils. Move your awareness up to your hip area and consciously relax your hips and the lower abdominal area. Breathe into your abdomen, relaxing your abdomen with your breath.

4. Now move up to your chest area and relax your upper chest, your back, spine, shoulders, arms, and hands. Feel the tingling sensation in these areas.

5. Move up to the neck and relax your neck muscles. Move to your head area and relax your entire head, your chin, cheeks, ears, nose, and eyes. Allow the mouth to relax by letting your jaw fall open. Relax your tongue. Remember to continue breathing through your nostrils. Relax your forehead, the back of your head, and the very top of the head.

6. Your entire body is now completely relaxed. You are lying completely still. You feel a warm, tingling sensation flowing through your entire body.

7. Continue lying in the Relaxation Posture for 10 breaths.

## Polarity Breath

The Polarity Breath allows you to drop one level deeper as you visualize yourself inhaling through one part of your body and exhaling through another. As you breathe in, feel the coolness of your breath as it enters your body, and feel the coolness of the breath as it leaves. With each exhalation, your body becomes softer and softer. You feel safer and safer. The safer you feel inside your body, the more you will be able to let go. The more you can let go, the more relaxed you become and the more benefit you will receive from the postures. As you shift your attention from one side of your body to the other in this breathing exercise, you balance your male and female energies within.

1. Continue to lie in the Relaxation Posture. Focus your attention to the bottom of your right foot. When you inhale, breathe in as if breathing through the bottom of that foot. Shift your consciousness to the palm of your left hand. When you exhale, exhale as if exhaling through the palm of your left hand. Continue this for 5 breaths, inhaling from the bottom of your right foot, exhaling through the palm of your left hand.

2. On your next inhalation, shift your consciousness to the bottom of your left foot. Draw in your breath from the bottom of your left foot and exhale through the palm of your right hand. As you continue to do the Polarity Breath, allow your lips to part and your jaw to open. Your entire body is relaxed. Continue this for 5 more breaths.

3. On your next breath, breathe in through the bottoms of both feet, and exhale through the palms of both hands. Continue breathing this way for 5 more breaths.

4. On your next breath, continue breathing in from the bottoms of both feet, drawing the breath all the way up your spine and out through the top of your head. Feel the breath leaving the top of your head, allowing any tension to leave the body. Continue exhaling through the top of your head for 5 more breaths.

5. In the next breath, lift your hands over your head and stretch your body. Make noises and sounds. Your body likes to release through sound. Twist and turn. Feel the energy release any deeper tension.

## Abdominal Breath

The purpose of this breathing exercise is to further relax your body and to release negative feelings and/or blockages trapped inside the body. Reclaim the natural rhythm of your breath. Feel it. You are unique. Listen to your own body to find its unique rhythm of breathing. The next breath becomes deeper. As you focus on the Abdominal Breath, feel your abdominal cavity being worked, releasing stress in the body.

1. Lie in the Relaxation Posture and breathe through your nostrils. Focus your attention on your abdomen, and when you inhale, fill your abdomen up like a balloon, bringing in oxygen. (See Figure 4-3.)

2. When you exhale, squeeze your abdomen into your spine. Press your abdominal muscles and lower back into the floor, squeezing all the air out. The next breath becomes deeper. (See Figure 4-4.)

3. As you focus on the Abdominal Breath, your body becomes more and more relaxed. Consciously walk your shoulders down from your ears and continue to do the Abdominal Breath. Allow your breath to be smooth and even. Breathe in and out, continuing the Abdominal Breath for 10 more breaths.

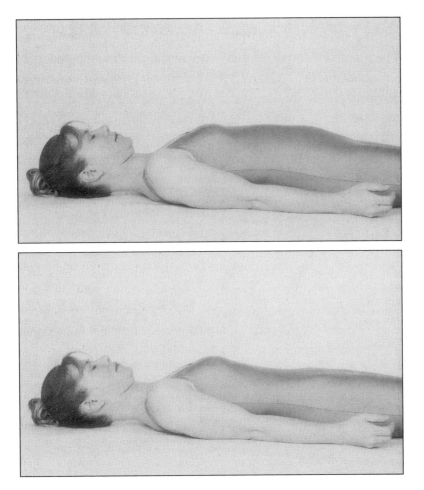

**Figure 4-3**
*Inhale and fill your abdomen up like a balloon, bringing in oxygen, filling up all the way.*

**Figure 4-4**
*Exhale and squeeze all the air out, pressing your abdominal muscles into your spine.*

## Alternate Nostril Breath (*Anuloma Viloma*)

The Alternate Nostril Breath is wonderful for cleansing on a physical and mental level. Physically, this breathing exercise clears your head, relieving tension headaches, clearing sinuses or a runny or congested nasal passage. You clear the nasal passage with your breath. This breathing exercise is also an excellent way to help expand your lung capacity.

On an emotional level, the Alternate Nostril Breath cleanses you as it clears and relaxes your mind, leaving you feeling refreshed and mentally alert. Holding your breath during this exercise allows you to pause, teaching you to pause in life. It gives your mind a chance to slow down, helping you to put things into perspective.

1. Come into a comfortable sitting position. Close your eyes and begin breathing through your nostrils while you place your hands on your knees, palms up. Adjust any part of your body that needs adjusting, ensuring your spine is straight to allow for a flow of energy along the spine.

2. With your right hand, take your fourth finger and place it on the outside of your left nostril. Breathe in slowly from your right nostril for a count of 8. (See Figure 4-5.)

3. Now squeeze both nostrils with your thumb and fourth finger, and hold your breath for a count of 8. (See Figure 4-6.)

4. Lift the fourth finger from the nostril and slowly exhale for a count of 8 while depressing the right nostril with the thumb. (See Figure 4-7.) It is important to inhale and exhale slowly during this breathing exercise so as not to use up all your air too quickly.

*continued*

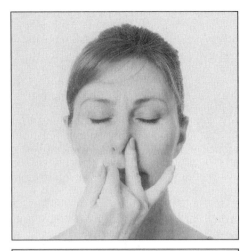

**Figure 4-5**

*Place your fourth finger on the outside of your left nostril and slowly breathe in through your right nostril.*

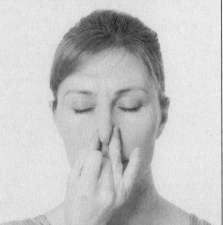

**Figure 4-6**

*Squeeze both nostrils using your thumb and fourth finger.*

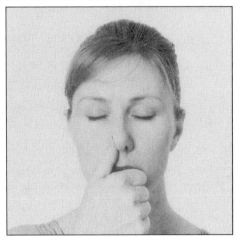

**Figure 4-7**

*Slowly exhale through your left nostril while depressing only the right nostril with your thumb.*

5. Now alternate sides, breathing in through your left nostril for a count of 8, holding your breath for a count of 8 while squeezing both nostrils, and exhaling for a count of 8 as you lift your thumb. This is one complete cycle.

6. Continue this breathing for 5 complete cycles, alternating the nostrils you use to inhale and exhale.

You may change the amount of time allotted for inhaling, holding, and exhaling to a time limit that better suits your lung capacity. Try inhaling, holding, and exhaling for a count of 6. Or, try a pattern of 4–8–16. Do whatever feels most comfortable for you. I find using the count of 8 the most comfortable. Using a set amount of time is following a structured pattern and is the disciplined approach to this exercise. Feel free to set up a non-structured time limit by inhaling, holding, and exhaling according to your own comfort level.

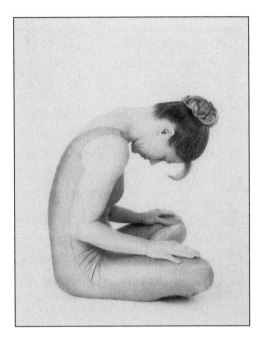

## Complete Breath

The Complete Breath is designed to increase the air capacity of your lungs. Pushing your hands into your knees allows the chest and lungs to open further so that more air can be taken in. Breathe slowly to help the lungs expand fully yet gently. Slowly exhale as you roll your head and upper body down, completely emptying your body of air.

1. Come into a comfortable sitting position with your legs crossed in front of you. Place the palms of your hands on your knees. Adjust any part of your body that needs adjusting, ensuring that your spine is straight to allow an energy flow through the spine.

2. Inhale and drop your chin to your chest, slowly rolling your head and shoulders down along with your spine. Exhale and squeeze the oxygen out of your abdomen. (See Figure 4-8.)

*continued*

**Figure 4-9**

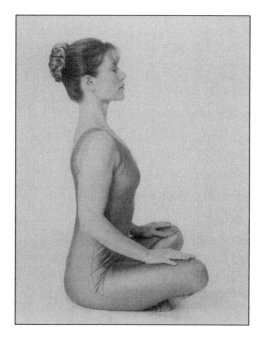

3. On your next inhalation, begin lifting the upper body slowly, filling your chest and abdomen with air as you inhale. Push your hands into your knees to help straighten your body more, opening the lungs and chest area further so that they may be filled with more air. (See Figure 4-9.)

4. Slowly exhale once again as you roll your head and upper body down, completely emptying your body of air. This is one complete cycle.

5. Continue this breath for 5 complete cycles of inhaling and exhaling.

## Chapter 5

# Visualization and Meditation

The Opening to Postures Visualization can be used after your pranayamas and just prior to entering your asanas, or postures. It is used to help get you more in tune to your "whole" body, bringing in an awareness of your body and mind and spirit, preparing your body for the postures. Before beginning your postures, tell yourself you are taking an inner journey of love and nurturing, consciously setting aside the stresses of the day.

The Closing Meditation can be used to end your yoga program, to allow the body some time to relax as well as to allow for the body/mind integration to occur once the postures are performed.

Follow the full Chakra Mediation when doing your breathing exercises, as part of your daily meditation, to help keep you open and balanced emotionally. This meditation can also be used before entering your postures, opening all your chakras at once, and then enjoying a free flow of postures as your body dictates.

## Opening to Postures Visualization

Come into a comfortable sitting or lying position. Close your eyes and begin breathing through your nostrils. As you sit, honor your body—your physical, emotional, and mental body. Begin with your physical body, then move into your emotional and mental body.

Become aware of your posture. Scan your body—your physical body. Thank it for serving you and being healthy. Now, scan your physical body to find if any part of your body is uncomfortable. Stay in your center, your still point, and scan. Acknowledge any discomfort.

Allow yourself a few minutes to complete scanning your physical body.

Now move to your emotional body. Thank it for serving you the best it can. Pay attention to the feelings that come up as you honor your feeling body.

*"I feel . . . ."*

It doesn't need to be a lot of words. Do not monitor or judge yourself. Take a few minutes to honor your emotional body by acknowledging how you feel.

Take in another deep breath and move into your mental body.

Thank your mental body for serving you and that you know it is serving you to the best of its ability. You want to capture the thought of the moment, what is happening in your mind.

*"My thoughts are . . . ."*

Acknowledge these thoughts as real, taking a few minutes as you honor your mental body.

Now that you have emptied and acknowledged all the parts of your self, know you automatically draw in your spiritual body. Your spiritual body is also known as your higher self. As you draw in your higher self, you will be guided from a higher place as you go through your postures.

## Closing Meditation

End your yoga program with the following meditation. As mentioned in chapter 3, it is always important to follow your postures with a few minutes of relaxation, allowing your body the chance to assimilate what it has learned. Be aware that as you perform your postures, you not only release on a physical level, but on an emotional and mental level as well. Relaxation helps create a space for healing, and gives you that quiet moment needed to acknowledge your growth.

> Come into the Relaxation Posture (Figure 4-2, page 23) so that you can relax your entire body. Focus once again on your breath, breathing in and out through your nostrils, bringing your awareness back inside to your center, to that place where we nurture our bodies.

> Fill your lungs with oxygen, filling up all the way, allowing your breath to calm your mind, to still the mind.

> As you breathe in, imagine breathing in a white light, filling up all the spaces—your head, your neck, your shoulders, arms, hands and fingers, your torso, your hips, your legs, feet, and toes—so that now your entire body is filled with this white light, allowing your inner light to shine brightly.

> Take a moment to step back now, to be in the stillness of your own being. As you do this, you balance. Allow yourself to breathe deeply. Take some time to be with yourself. You may find yourself drifting off. This is okay. Allow yourself to trust what is happening—the body/mind integration. You are aware you are in a very safe place.

> Now, create a silent moment for yourself. Transport yourself near some water—a river or a lake. See yourself lying there in the sun. Ask the rays to be on you, feeling their warmth. You can feel the sand and hear the water. Allow your feelings to come out, knowing you are taken care of. Your needs will always be met. Take a moment to acknowledge these wonderful things and how far you

have come. Acknowledge this with gratitude and then allow a period of quiet to take place so that you may grow.

As you finish your journey, allow yourself to stay in tune to your body and your needs. Know you have access to new knowledge, and that you can bring this knowledge into your daily life whenever needed. Make a commitment to stay centered and focused for the rest of the day. Breathe. You are experiencing a sense of calm. Know you can draw on this source of strength and peacefulness whenever needed, never leaving your center.

Allow yourself some time to sit in silence and your inner light to shine brighter in the silence. When you're ready, slowly come back.

Stretch your body so that you are fully back. Take your time.

## Chakra Meditation

### For Opening and Balancing the Chakras

Come into a comfortable sitting or lying position, whichever is most comfortable for you, and begin breathing through your nostrils. Allow your spine to be as straight as possible to allow for an energy flow through your body. Close your eyes and continue breathing through your nostrils, completely filling your lungs with air. When you exhale, completely empty the air out of your lungs. This is not an exaggerated breath. Breathe calmly and slowly, taking about twenty of these slow, connected breaths into your lungs. Follow your breath, and as you do, you begin to feel stress and tension leaving your body. Your body is becoming completely relaxed and calm. You feel a sense of stillness surround you.

Allow your awareness to fall to the very base of your spine, to your tailbone. You see a beautiful ruby red color. This is your first chakra, known as your Root chakra. Place a band of ruby red both in the front and behind your tailbone, visualizing it surrounding your spine, rotating in a clockwise direction. As you breathe in the red, affirm to yourself:

*"I am safe and secure."*

Activate the vibration of the color so that you can begin to feel the quality of the affirmation. The Root chakra has to do with your feelings of security, confidence, and survival. It is a grounding energy that has to do with how comfortable you feel in your body, learning to break away from societal beliefs and feeling comfortable for doing so.

Move up to your lower abdomen now, to your second chakra, your Sacral chakra. You see a wonderful deep orange surrounding your spine from a spot directly above your tailbone to a point approximately 2 inches below your navel. As you breathe in this wonderful orange color, affirm to yourself:

*"I create with love. That I was created from love. I create with abundance not fear. When I create with love I am in the flow of God's gifts."*

This chakra is known as your Creative center, your center for creative and sexual energy. The body parts of this chakra include your hips, as well as your sex organs, uterus, and womb, the area in which you were created. It has to do with your relationship to others and how you relate to them on a one-to-one basis.

The second chakra is also known as your Abundance center. As you create out of love, you create abundance in your life. Breathe in the orange. As you do, draw in whatever you need to feel comfortable in life.

Move up to your third chakra now, your Solar Plexus chakra. You see a bright sunshine yellow. Place a band of sunshine yellow in the front and behind your spine, from the spot 2 inches above your navel all the way up to your rib cage. This center is also known as your Power center as well as your Emotional center because this is where you house your power and your emotions. It can also be referred to as your Action center as you learn to act out your emotions. Breathe in the sunshine yellow and affirm to yourself:

*"I trust my feelings and am at peace in my power center. I trust my feelings."*

This is where you feel your feelings, knowing that in order to stay balanced and healthy you must learn to express them. This chakra has to do with your relationship to self.

As you move up to your fourth chakra, your Heart chakra, you see a beautiful emerald green. Place a band of emerald green in front and behind your Heart center, all the way up to your throat, covering your chest, your back and shoulders down your arms, hands and fingers. Your Heart chakra is "knowing." You are in the middle now, the halfway point, the center for forgiveness and compassion and the center of your humanness, where you learn your lessons. This energy center reminds you of giving and receiving love. Look into your Heart and feel the balancing. Feel how love heals. You are in the middle. Pause here before entering the denser, more physical energies below or the lighter, more spiritual energies above. Breathe in the emerald green and affirm:

*"My heart is open."*

Know that to experience what it means to be "fully" human, you must experience both the higher, more spiritual energies above your Heart chakra as well as the lower, more denser energies below it.

As you move up to your fifth chakra, your Throat chakra, you see a clear sky blue color. Place a band of sky blue in the front and behind your Throat chakra, from the base of your throat all the way up to just below the eyebrows, covering your neck, your entire face, your chin, the cheeks, eyes, nose, and ears. Your eyes are included in your Throat chakra because your eyes express the emotion of what your throat is saying. As you breathe in the sky blue, affirm to yourself:

*"I speak the truth; I speak freely; my throat is open."*

To speak your truth, use discernment. Speak your feelings, but first by passing through your Heart chakra. This is why the Heart chakra is placed where it is. You speak without disempowering. The Throat chakra teaches you to be responsive rather than reactive—learning to step back and pause, and to come from your heart.

Move up to your sixth chakra now, your Third Eye, located at your forehead area.

You see a bright indigo blue. Place a band of indigo blue in the front and behind your forehead area, from a point above your eyebrows all the way up to the top of your head. Affirm to yourself:

*"I am intuitive."*

It is here that you access your intuition, that sense of knowing and trusting. You learn to come from living in the moment. Living in the moment takes the stress out of your life because you no longer have to fear what happened in the past or what may happen in the future. Living in the moment. Trusting the moment. When you do you are able to come from your higher mind.

Now move up to your Crown chakra, to the top of your head, where you see a violet purple light. Imagine the violet purple light swirling at the top of your head. Your Crown chakra is your higher self connection, your connection to God, and to spirit.

Breathing in through the Crown at the top of your head puts you immediately in touch to your higher self and to spirit. Affirm:

*"I am a being of pure light."*

It is here that we recognize we are pure beings. The Crown chakra is your energy vortex. You can see your soul star above your Crown chakra. Knowledge comes through your soul star, into your Crown, and down through the rest of your chakras.

When all your chakras are open and the colors of the rainbow are aligned in the spine, their colors resonate the color white. Imagine your body filling up with this white color, filling up all the spaces in your body, your arms and fingers, your head and neck, the hip and abdominal area, legs, and feet. Fill your body with this white light. Feel its warmth. Lie in your stillness for a few moments as your body radiates this warm, white light.

Slowly begin to come back. Allow yourself to sit in silence for a few moments, feeling completely balanced, your inner light shining brighter as you slowly come back.

Now is a good time to move into your postures, now that you are open and have begun to release.

# Chapter 6

# Asanas

Asanas are the heart of your yoga program. They are the gentle stretches and postures used in yoga to exert your physical body with the intent to add strength, stamina, and flexibility. They are also meant to leave you feeling energized and invigorated, helping to maintain a heightened awareness of your body. Just one session of a few key postures can erase any kinks, aches, or pains I may wake up with on a given day. I am always amazed at the magical effect yoga has on my body.

As with other physical fitness programs, yoga uses static and isometric motion as you enter a posture slowly and carefully, stretching the muscles in use and then comfortably holding the position for a few breaths. Doing the postures in this manner helps to build long, lean, and limber muscles. Being aware of where you are placing the different parts of your body allows you to position yourself safely and properly. Holding the posture strengthens your physical body and gives you a chance to feel how you respond to the posture, both physically and emotionally.

Yoga is not considered to be an aerobic activity. However, you will receive some aerobic benefit and cardiovascular conditioning from the postures as your stamina increases and as you advance through your yoga program, practicing the postures in a rhythmic flow. An aerobic activity is any non-stop activity that uses the large muscle groups, such as your legs and hips. Using these muscles through constant motion promotes cardiovascular fitness and endurance. As you work these muscles, your oxygen intake increases and an increased supply of blood is sent to the heart, making the heart work harder and become stronger. As the heart becomes stronger, more oxygen reaches the blood. You will notice your heart working harder with many of the postures such as the Extended Triangle, any of the heart chakra postures (Chakra Four postures), and the Sun Salutation.

Although modern-day yoga's focus is primarily on postures to build physical fitness, chakra yoga focuses on practicing all areas of Sadhana, as explained in chapter 3. The keystone behind chakra yoga is that the physical body is connected to the emotional and/or mental body. Working your physical body through postures can help you work through issues that have settled in your emotional and/or mental body. Your awareness of being able to experience emotional feelings through the postures, and also by acknowledging these feelings, will aid you in letting them go if you feel they no longer serve your highest good.

In chakra yoga, you work your physical, mental, and emotional bodies. Physically, you add strength, stamina, and flexibility. Emotionally and mentally, you open your awareness to these aspects of yourself—calming your mind and releasing stress and negative feelings and blockages. I practice my yoga by separating the postures by chakra and this is how I have written this book. Understanding the postures by chakra is how I was taught yoga, and so it makes sense to me to practice it this way. I am able to derive more benefit as I am aware of which emotional body I am activating, as I work myself physically and tap into myself emotionally.

As you will learn, your chakras, or energy centers, relate directly to your physical body. Structuring the postures by chakra ensures that each part of your body has been used. During your own yoga program, there will be time to complete 2 to 3 postures per chakra before moving on to the next chakra. As you move up along the spine to each new chakra location, you become one with that chakra.

My yoga instructor, Fazia Khan, taught me to follow a meditation before entering each new chakra, in order to activate the energy within. This helps the chakra to continue to open and balance as you engage in the postures that correspond to the body parts of that area. Through the postures, you will innately learn what each chakra has to teach you and how they are meant to help you. I have included a brief meditation at the start of each chakra's postures to help you activate each chakra as you enter it. By taking this important step of "going within" to focus on the chakra before performing its postures, Fazia taught me the inner beauty and gentleness yoga has to offer. I acknowledge this with gratitude and that much of what I pass on to you in these meditations is from the knowledge passed on to me through Fazia's teachings and her incredible insight.

Organizing the postures by chakra helps you to focus and concentrate on the area of the body that is being worked. You become aware of the body parts that should and should not be used in a particular posture as you focus on entering and completing a posture properly and without injury.

This system also ensures that no part of the body has been missed. Of course, when creating your own yoga program, you can choose which postures to do to meet your own individual needs. If you think you need extra work on strengthening the abdominals, concentrate on the Chakra Three postures. If you need to alleviate pain or tightness in the neck area, concentrate on the Chakra Five postures.

Organizing the postures by chakra will also allow you to easily locate which postures you want to do simply by knowing which area of your body needs to be worked. As you pass through each chakra, you learn what is holding you back emotionally. When you are able to recognize and feel this, you then know what area to work on to release those blockages. This is how you strengthen your physical, emotional, and mental body to overcome weaknesses.

Another approach my students often prefer is to go through a complete meditation to open all their chakras at once and then enjoy a free flow of postures without interruption. I have inserted the full Chakra

Meditation in chapter 5 so that you too can try this approach, moving from one posture to the next as your body dictates. Keeping centered and in tune to what your body needs is how you derive the most from your daily yoga program.

So, to recap, your postures can be performed by chakra, opening each chakra first with the brief meditation inserted at the beginning of each chakra's postures, or by going into a free flow of postures, as your body dictates, by first opening all your chakras through the full Chakra Mediation.

A beginner can safely do most of the postures demonstrated in the book. Always remember to listen to your body and only go into a posture as far as your comfort level permits. Go at your own pace. Do only the postures with which you are comfortable. After a few weeks, you will notice your body is able to stretch further into the postures. Allow your body to advance naturally, at its own pace. I have demonstrated the advanced positions of each posture as they apply, allowing you to advance as your body permits, when your body is ready. These are the goals you are working toward as you progress gently with your yoga.

The postures I include in this book are those I feel give you the most benefit. They are all considered to be "foundation" or basic postures. I have included some variations, however, I suggest you do not stray too far from the position of a foundation posture as this is usually the one offering the most benefit. I have included a variation only if it is safe, adds further benefit, or works another set of muscles without added strain to the back or neck.

I am not a proponent of practicing a posture only because it looks good. Some postures can cause more harm than good if not performed properly. I have not included any variations to postures that put unnecessary strain on your body. Be assured the postures demonstrated provide ample variety to create your own program that will best suit your needs.

When creating a program, try and choose 2 to 3 postures from each chakra to ensure every muscle in your body has been exercised. On the days that certain parts of your body need more attention, do the postures that apply to those areas.

For variety, try opening your chakras through the full Chakra Meditation, and then continue on with a free flow of postures, flowing smoothly from one posture to the next without interruption. Again, it is up to you to decide how you choose to create your yoga program. Some days you may want to organize your postures by chakra, helping your focus remain on the body part being worked. Other days you may enjoy a free flow of postures, innately performing postures as your body dictates.

For your convenience, at the end of this chapter, I have suggested three yoga programs for you to follow as a start. As you advance through your yoga and become more in tune with your body and more familiar with the postures, you will be able to fine-tune a program to better suit your individual needs.

As mentioned, there are several postures not included in this book simply because I feel they pose too much strain on your body, especially the lower back and neck. For an inclusive source of postures, consult your local library or bookstore for other yoga books.

You are now ready to begin the postures. Remember, it is always important to begin your program with relaxation and breathing exercises as well as to end your postures with a few minutes of relaxation. This allows the body to assimilate what it has learned—"the body/mind integration." (See chapter 4 for relaxation and breathing exercises and chapter 5 for the Closing Meditation.)

Some personal reminders before I close:

- Be gentle on yourself. Don't expect too much or give up when you feel frustrated. Your muscles have a memory, and your flexibility and coordination will come back. It may take time, so be patient.

- Remember to breathe throughout each posture. Breathing will make all the difference in getting you through a posture. If, at times, you are not able to do a certain posture, check to see if you are breathing properly before giving up. Chances are you are holding your breath, making the posture more difficult to complete.

- Whenever possible, completely let yourself go. Open your heart and your mind. Completely surrender yourself, especially when holding a position, so that you can experience the beauty, gentleness, and grace in yoga. As you allow yourself to do this, you begin the process of letting go of those things that no longer feel comfortable in your body.

Chapter 7

# Starting Positions

Beginning your postures properly is one of the most important things you can do for yourself when following a yoga program at home on your own. Getting into the posture too quickly, or skipping important steps, can cause strain, followed by stiffness, to the muscles being used, as well as strain or even injury to muscles that should not be in use as a result of not entering the posture properly.

As explained earlier, it is important to enter a posture slowly and carefully, being aware of where you are to place your body parts, allowing you to position yourself safely and properly. Take your time. Begin by closing your eyes and focusing inward for a few breaths, breathing in and out through your nostrils. Focus on the posture you are about to enter, paying particular attention to the muscles you are about to engage. Always begin your posture with the proper body alignment, always keeping your neck in alignment to your spine, concentrating only on the muscle and body parts about to be used, relaxing those that will not be involved.

Ensure that you continue breathing through your nostrils throughout the entire posture, never holding your breath. Sending oxygen to the muscles being used helps these muscles to release further into the posture, allowing them to become more flexible. Breathing during your postures will also prevent cramping during the postures, and/or dizziness that can often follow when holding your breath while holding the posture. Holding your breath during the postures can also cause stiffness in your muscles the next day.

The following are seven basic "starting" positions used to begin many of the postures in the book (usually described in step 1). Study these basic positions before beginning your yoga program.

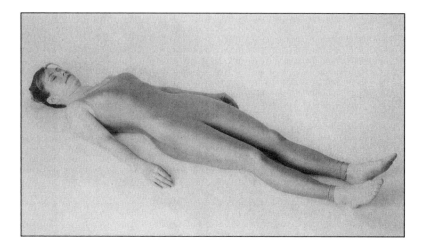

**Figure 7-1**
*Lie flat with your arms at your side, relaxing your neck and shoulders.*

## Lying Position

1. Lie on your back on the floor. Your feet are extended straight out in front of you. Your arms are at your sides, palms down. Your head is in alignment with your spine. Relax your neck and shoulders. Begin breathing through your nostrils. (See Figure 7-1.)

**Figure 7-2**
*Press your lower back
into the floor to help
support your spine.*

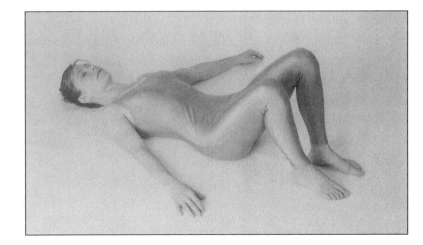

## Lying Position with Knees Bent

1. Lie on your back and bend your knees, placing your
   feet on the floor. Press your lower back into the floor.
   Your arms are at your sides, palms down. Your head is
   in alignment with your spine. Relax your neck and
   shoulders. Begin breathing through your nostrils.
   (See Figure 7-2.)

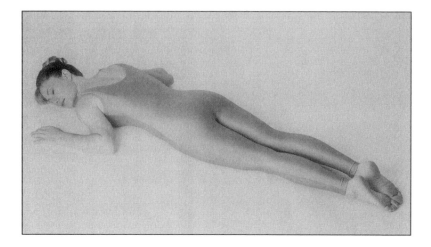

**Figure 7-3**
*Place your head to one side to help relax your neck.*

## Tummy Position

1. Lie on your tummy (abdomen) and place your head to one side to relax your neck. Your arms are out to the sides, palms down. Your legs are extended out comfortably, feet together. Begin breathing through your nostrils. (See Figure 7-3.)

**Figure 7-4**

*Make sure you are comfortable as you cross your legs and sit up as straight as possible.*

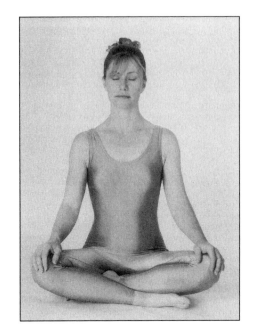

## Comfortable Sitting Position (*Sukhasana*)

1.  Sit on the floor and cross your legs. Make sure you are comfortable. Sit up as straight as you can with your head resting comfortably between your shoulders. Your neck is in alignment with your spine. Your arms and hands are resting on your knees. Relax your neck and shoulders. Begin breathing through your nostrils. (See Figure 7-4.)

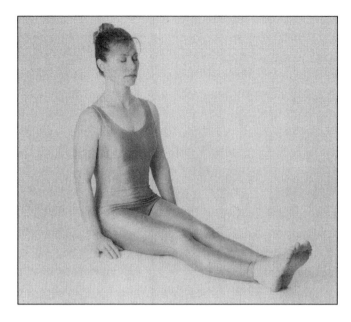

**Figure 7-5**
*Relax your neck and shoulders as you sit up as straight as you can while keeping your legs straight.*

## Sitting Position with Legs Extended

1. Sit on the floor, extending your legs out in front of you. Keep your legs as straight as possible as you sit up as straight as you can. Your head is resting comfortably between your shoulders. Your neck is in alignment with your spine. Your arms and hands are at the sides of your body, palms down. Relax your neck and shoulders. Begin breathing through your nostrils. (See Figure 7-5.)

### Comfort Aid
*If you have difficulty sitting up straight, sit on two or three towels or folded blankets, supporting your thighs.*

*If you find your back is weak, sit up against a wall with a towel or cushion behind your waist or chest.*

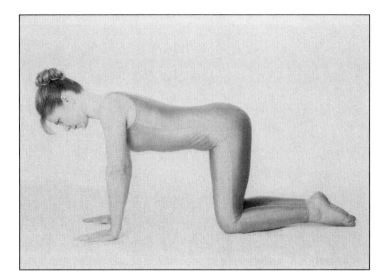

## Table Position

1. Come up onto all fours with your hands and knees placed shoulder width apart. Your back should be completely flat. Your head and neck are in alignment with your spine. Begin breathing through your nostrils. (See Figure 7-6.)

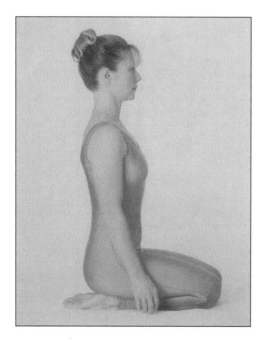

**Figure 7-7**
*Sit up as straight as you can while sitting on your feet.*

## Kneeling Position

1. Kneel on the floor, sitting on your feet. Your arms are at your side. Sit up as straight as you can with your head resting comfortably between your shoulders. Your neck is in alignment with your spine. Begin breathing through your nostrils. (See Figure 7-7.)

### Comfort Aid

*If you have difficulty sitting on your feet, place a soft blanket or towel under your feet for added cushioning. Or place the towel between your buttocks and feet to help relieve the pressure on your shins/feet.*

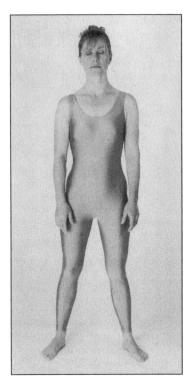

**Figure 7-8**

*Squeeze your buttocks to help support the spine. Keep your knees in a slightly unlocked position to take any strain off your lower back.*

## Standing Position

1.  Stand with your feet shoulder width apart. Your arms are at your sides. You are standing as straight as you can with your head resting comfortably between your shoulders. Your neck is in alignment with your spine. Relax your neck and shoulders. Squeeze your buttocks and keep your knees in a slightly unlocked position. Begin breathing through your nostrils. (See Figure 7-8.)

## Chapter 8

# Limbering Up

You are now ready to begin your postures. Start your program with a few gentle stretches to help warm and limber up your muscles. This sends the message to your body that it is about to be worked on, preparing it for asanas. As in any exercise program, taking the time to warm up your muscles increases the circulation of blood to the muscles, making them more flexible. It is especially important if you choose to do your yoga in the morning, when the muscles are generally a little more stiff. It may help to have a warm shower or bath before starting to help warm up and loosen tightness, allowing you to stretch further into the postures.

Choose 3 or 4 of these postures to practice before starting your yoga program. Keep in mind these postures can also be used within your yoga program whenever you feel the need to loosen up further. Try and keep your eyes closed, always remembering to breathe through your nostrils throughout the postures.

## Knee to Chest Posture

We hold a lot of tension in the hip and lower back area. This posture will help your body to begin releasing built-up tension. You will feel the stretch predominately in the lower back, but by keeping both shoulders on the floor, you will feel a gentle stretch along the entire spine as well.

1. Come into a lying position with your legs extended. Bend your right knee into your chest and gently press it down. (See Figure 8-1.) Consciously relax your neck and shoulders and continue breathing through your nose.

2. Press your lower back into the floor as you continue to press your knee into your abdomen. Hold for 5 breaths, limbering up the hip area.

3. Slide your right leg down next to your left leg and shake both legs out.

4. Repeat the same sequence with your left leg.

5. Now press both knees into your chest and continue inhaling through your nostrils. (See Figure 8-2.)

6. With your arms straight out to the sides, rotate your lower body from side to side, massaging the lower back. Keep both shoulders on the floor and your feet together. Relax your upper body. (See Figure 8-3.)

7. Slide both legs down back into the lying position. Rest a moment while breathing through your nose.

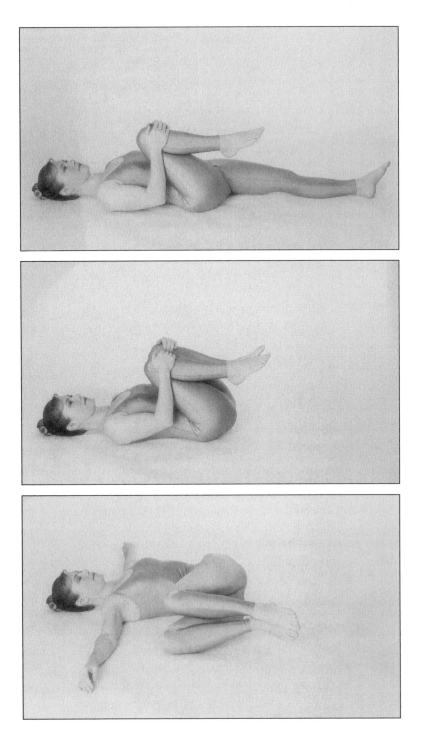

**Figure 8-1**

*Relax your neck and shoulders as you press your knee into your chest. Feel a gentle stretch in your thigh and buttock area.*

**Figure 8-2**

*Press your lower back into the floor as you press both knees into your chest.*

**Figure 8-3**

*Massage your lower back as you rotate your knees from side to side. Feel the stretch along your spine, mostly in your lower back.*

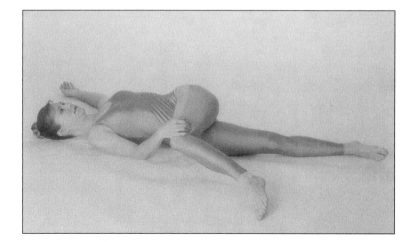

## Knee Down Twist

This posture gives a nice twist and stretch to your lower back, and a deeper stretch to your spine as you swing one leg over the opposite hip area. Feel the tension being released as you twist and stretch your spine. You may hear the release in the form of a crack. Do not be alarmed. This is okay.

1. Come into a lying position. Bend your left knee into your chest, keeping your right leg fully extended on the floor. Gently press your knee into your chest with both hands.

2. Exhale and swing your left knee over the right hip. Both shoulders remain on the floor. Relax your neck, shoulders, and entire back and gently press down on your left knee with your right hand. Your knee does not have to touch the floor. (See Figure 8-4.) Breathe into the lower back to help relax the muscles, releasing any tension in the lower back. Hold this position for 5 breaths.

3. Swing your knee back over and slide the leg down to meet the right leg. Shake both legs out and pause for a moment, continuing to breathe through the nostrils.

4. Repeat this sequence with your right leg.

## Counter Posture

Bend both knees into the chest to help release the lower back, and slide the legs back down into the lying position.

## Ankle to Knee Posture

**Extra Help**

When extending your leg, bend your knee as much as is necessary. Work toward straightening the leg.

This posture is a gentle stretch used to release the hip area. You will feel a deeper stretch in the hip and groin area as you extend and straighten the bent leg.

1. Come into a lying position with your knees bent. Place your right ankle on your left knee. Gently press down on the right knee with your right hand for 5 breaths. Send your breath to your hip area. (See Figure 8-5.)

2. Extend your left leg, straightening it as much as possible. Grab your left calf as you lift your left leg, keeping the right ankle on the left knee. Gently press your left leg into your chest for 5 breaths, holding onto the calf or wherever it is comfortable. (See Figure 8-6.)

3. Lower your left foot down to the floor, then your right leg. Repeat steps 1 and 2 with your left leg.

4. Slide both legs down to the floor into the lying position.

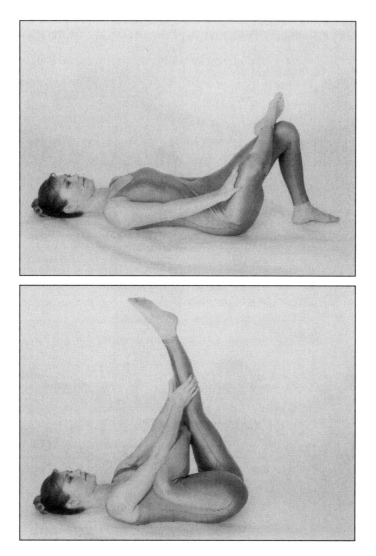

**Figure 8-5**
*Gently press down on your knee to help loosen up the hip area.*

**Figure 8-6**
*Feel the stretch in the hip, hamstrings, and groin area as you extend and gently press your leg toward your chest. Try not to pull your leg with your hands.*

# Pelvic Rock into Pelvic Tilt (*Urdhva Dhanurasana*)

This posture is used to awaken the energy in your pelvis and hip area. When in the Pelvic Rock, let your body feel when it wants to rest before going into the Pelvic Tilt. Squeezing your buttocks as you lift yourself into the tilt will help the body be lifted further. Remember to relax the upper body, neck, and shoulders as you lift your hips and press them into the ceiling.

1. Come into a lying position with your knees bent and arms out to the sides. Relax your upper body.

2. Locate your pelvis and gently rock the lower back and pelvic area along the spine, back and forth, without leaving the floor. Press the lower back into the floor as you roll up. (See Figure 8-7.) Now allow the lower back to arch up while you roll down. (See Figure 8-8.) This is the Pelvic Rock. Do this slowly and gently. Stop when you feel your body wanting to rest.

3. Inhale and lift your buttocks off the floor, transferring your weight onto your upper back. Squeeze your buttocks as you press your feet into the floor, allowing the body to be lifted further. Adjust your arms down along your body or wherever it is comfortable. This is the Pelvic Tilt. (See Figure 8-9.) Continue to relax your upper body, neck, and shoulders and continue to squeeze your buttocks as you press your hips square into the ceiling. Hold for 5 breaths.

4. For an added stretch, if you like, clasp your hands under your buttocks, squeezing your shoulder blades together. (See Figure 8-10, page 68.) Continue to press your feet into the floor as you lift your hips square into the ceiling. Hold for 5 breaths. Continue to squeeze your buttocks to protect your lower back.

*continued*

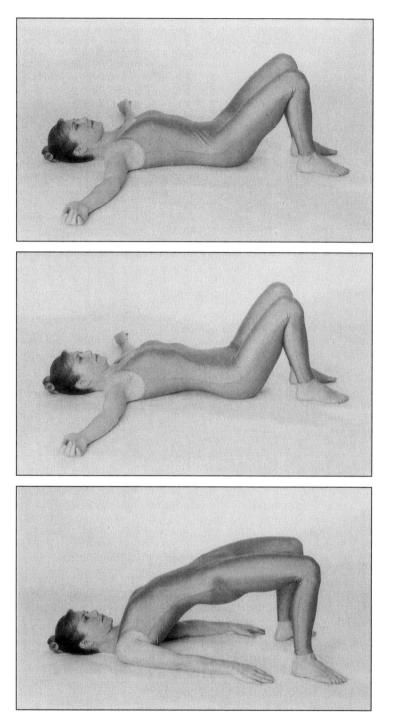

**Figure 8-7**
*The lower back is pressed into the floor as you roll up the pelvic area.*

**Figure 8-8**
*Notice the arch in the lower back as you roll down the pelvic area, pressing your tailbone into the floor. You are warming up the hip area as you rock up and down.*

**Figure 8-9**
*Feel the stretch in your thighs and up into the hips and lower back area as you lift up. Continue to squeeze your buttocks to protect your lower back.*

**Figure 8-10**

*For an added stretch in your upper back area, clasp your hands under your buttocks, squeezing your shoulder blades together.*

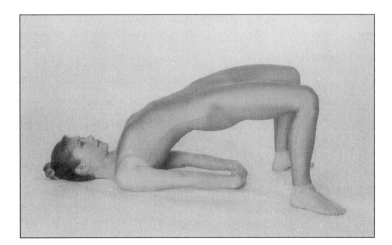

**Figure 8-11**

*For extra support during the Pelvic Tilt, place your hands on your buttocks or lower back.*

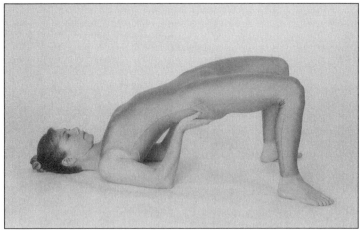

5. Lower your body down. Bring both knees into the chest and gently press down on them with your hands to release any tension in the lower back.

6. Slide your legs down into the Relaxation Posture (Figure 4-2, page 23). Breathe in and relax for a moment.

## Variation

During step 3, place the palms of your hands on your lower back or buttocks for extra support as you lift your buttocks. (See Figure 8-11.)

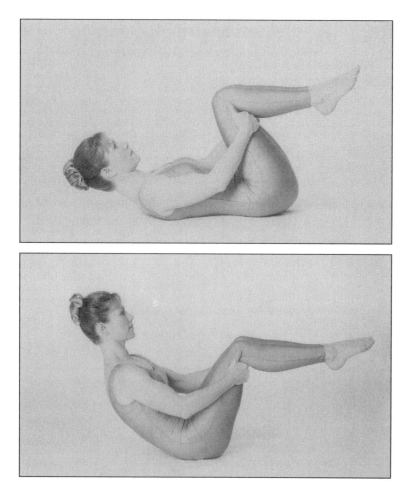

**Figure 8-12**
*Place your hands under your knees, lifting your head and neck off the floor.*

**Figure 8-13**
*Begin rocking back and forth, gaining momentum.*

## Spinal Rock

Use this posture to easily bring yourself into a sitting position from a lying position, without disrupting the flow of energy.

1. Come into a lying position. Bring both knees into your chest and place your hands under your knees, lifting your head and neck off the floor. (See Figure 8-12.)

2. Begin rocking your body back and forth by lifting your chest, then your abdominal muscles, as you push with your legs. (See Figure 8-13.) Continue rocking until you have gathered enough momentum to come into a sitting position. You are now ready to go into any sitting posture.

# Single Leg Extended Stretch (*Anantasana*)

This gently stretches the entire inside of your leg. Work toward keeping your leg as straight as possible throughout this stretch.

1. Come into a lying position. Turn to your right side, propping yourself up on your elbow. Bend your left knee into your chest, holding it with your left arm. (See Figure 8-14.)

2. Extend your left leg up as you grab hold of your calf or foot, wherever it is comfortable, keeping your leg as straight as possible. Gently pull the leg toward you to increase the stretch. (See Figure 8-15.) Point your toes for 5 breaths. Flex your toes for 5 breaths.

3. Lower your leg and rest for a few breaths.

4. Repeat, lying on your left side.

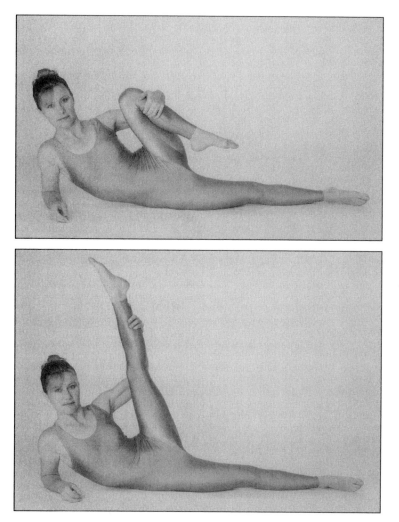

**Figure 8-14**
*Begin to feel a stretch in your hamstring and groin area as you hold your knee into your chest.*

**Figure 8-15**
*Feel a deeper stretch in the hamstrings, groin, and entire length of your raised leg as you gently pull it toward you.*

Chapter 9

# Stretching the Spine

There are not many forms of exercise that deal specifically with the spine, promoting the health of your spine. This is what makes yoga unique. The following postures are designed specifically for stretching and twisting the spine. In yoga, this is referred to as "awakening the spine." The stretching and twisting "awakens" the energy resting there and prepares your body to release once you are in the flow of postures. These gentle twists also gently squeeze your organs, squeezing toxins out, bringing in new blood and oxygen to your organs and cells.

The spine loves this attention. It is important for you to do this so that the muscles that surround and support the spine remain healthy and flexible. Your spine is the body's support system. Without keeping it healthy and limber, your body tightens and stiffens up. We cease to function properly. Even simple tasks become tiresome. Keeping these muscles healthy and flexible is imperative for a long and healthy life, serving to protect us well into our golden years.

Do these stretches between your postures whenever you feel the need to stretch your spine and/or the muscles surrounding it.

## Knee Down Twist

**Note**

*This posture is also used as a stretch in the "Limbering Up" postures in chapter 8.*

The Knee Down Twist gives a nice twist and stretch to your lower back, and a deeper stretch to your spine as you swing one leg over the opposite hip. Feel the tension being released as you twist and stretch your spine. You may hear the release in the form of a crack. Do not be alarmed. This is okay.

1. Come into a lying position. Bend your left knee into your chest, keeping your right leg fully extended on the floor. Gently press your knee into your chest with both hands.

2. Exhale and swing your left knee over the right hip area. Both shoulders remain on the floor. Relax your neck, shoulders, and entire back and gently press down on your left knee with your right hand. Your knee does not have to touch the floor. Breathe into the lower back to help relax the muscles, releasing any tension in the lower back. Hold for 5 breaths. (See Figure 8-4, page 62.)

3. Swing your knee back over and slide the leg down to meet the right leg. Shake both legs out and pause for a moment, continuing to breathe through the nostrils.

4. Repeat this sequence with your right leg.

### Counter Posture

Bend both knees into the chest to help release the lower back, and slide the legs back down into the lying position.

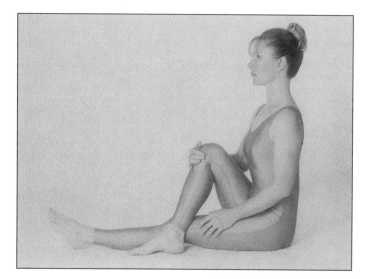

**Figure 9-1**
*Sit up as straight as you can as you place your right foot on the outside of your left knee.*

## Seated Spinal Twist (*Marichyasana*)

The Seated Spinal Twist allows you to stretch the entire length of your spine. As you engage your body in this stretch, consciously straighten your spine. Feel your chest open and expand as you do so. Breathe deeply into your chest, filling it with oxygen, and allowing the muscles along the spine to stretch further. You will also feel a stretch in your hips and upper back. This is a wonderful stretch for your spine. Notice how awake your body feels and how alert your mind has become.

1. Come into a seated position with your legs extended. Place your right foot on the outside of your left knee, flat on the floor. (See Figure 9-1.)

2. Grab your right foot with your right hand, placing your fingertips under your foot, if possible. Extend your left arm out in front of you. (See Figure 9-2, page 76.)

*continued*

**Figure 9-2**

*Grab your right foot with your right hand, placing your fingertips under your foot.*

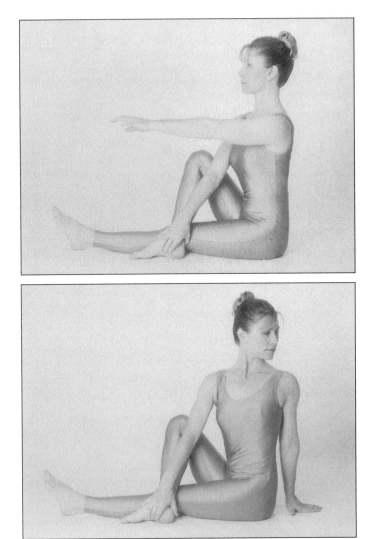

**Figure 9-3**

*Feel a stretch in your hips and upper back as you twist toward the back.*

3. Swing your left arm out to the side and all the way around to the back, keeping your arm straight. Place it as close to center back as is comfortable. Turn and follow your arm, engaging the spine in a twist. Breathe into the stretch to help relax the muscles. (See Figure 9-3.)

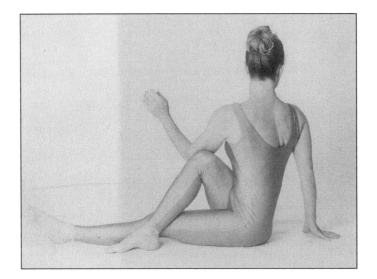

**Figure 9-4**
*For a counter stretch, place your left elbow on the outside of your right knee and twist to the right.*

4. Hold your body in this stretch for a count of 5 breaths, relaxing the neck and shoulders. Press the right foot into the floor. Sit up as straight as you can.

5. Release your left arm, lifting it up and swinging it around to the front of your body. The arm remains straight as you do this. Lower your arm down.

6. Release your right hand and extend both legs. Shake the legs out and pause for a moment.

7. Repeat the same sequence with your left leg.

## Variation

As you release your body from the twist and bring your extended arm back to the front (step 5), keep going and place your left elbow on the outside of the right knee. Extend your right hand to the side and turn your upper body 90 degrees. Keep your spine as straight as possible. (See Figure 9-4.)

*Focus*
*Remember to breathe to help relax the neck and shoulders as you stretch.*

*continued*

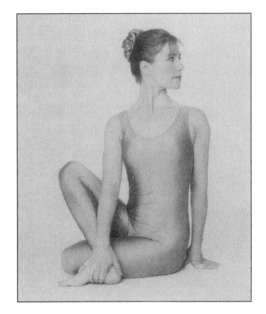

**Figure 9-5**

*For an added stretch in your thigh and hip area, tuck your left leg under as you twist.*

## Advanced

1. Coming from step 1, your right foot is placed on the outside of your left knee. Now tuck your left leg under your right leg, bending it back so that your left foot is placed as close to your right hip as is comfortable.

2. Twist to the left, placing your hand as close to center back as you can, progressing toward placing the palm flat on the floor. (See Figure 9-5.) Take your time, never pushing yourself further than your comfort level. Consciously send your breath to your lower arm where you feel the stretch, helping you reach into the stretch further.

## Standing Spinal Twist (*Marichyasana*)

Do this stretch after you have completed a standing posture. You will feel a stretch in the hips and upper thighs and along your entire spine and neck. Try to keep your eyes closed during this stretch as you focus on how your body feels.

1. Come into a standing position with your feet shoulder width apart. Stand as straight as you can. Extend both arms out in front and turn your upper body to the left. (See Figure 9-6, page 80.)

2. Lower your upper body to the floor, placing your right hand on the outside of your left foot. Straighten your legs as much as possible. Your left arm extends up as you turn and look behind. Straighten your left arm as much as you can and look up at your hand. (See Figure 9-7, page 80.) Hold this position for 5 breaths. Consciously relax your neck and shoulders as you breathe into the stretch.

3. Now come out of the posture the same way you came into it. Lift your upper body, coming back into a standing position. Your upper body is still facing to the left with both arms extended out. Swing the left arm back to center and lower both arms down to your sides as you breathe in and pause.

4. Repeat this sequence on the right side.

*continued*

**Focus**
*Bend your knees as much as necessary when placing your hands on the floor. Work toward straightening your legs.*

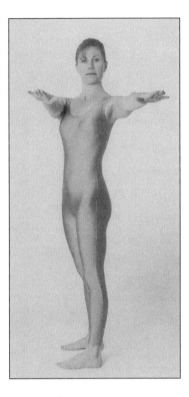 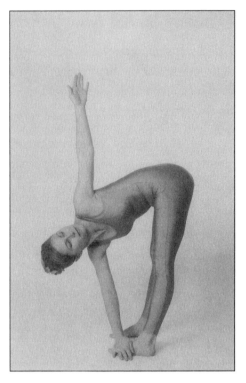

**Figure 9-6**

*Extend both arms out and turn your upper body to the left.*

**Figure 9-7**

*Straighten your left arm as much as you can and look up at your hand. Your palm is flat, fingers pointing up.*

## Alternate Table, Cat, and Dog Postures

The Table, Cat, and Dog are a series of movements that stretch the entire length of your spine. As you flow between the Cat and the Dog, you are reversing the arch in your spine, helping to release tightness and blocked energy resting there. The Table is a transition posture in this series, allowing your spine a chance to rest between alternating arches.

**Note**
*These poses are also used as counter postures.*

1. Bring yourself onto all fours, placing your palms and knees shoulder width apart. Your back and spine are completely flat in the Table position, with your neck in alignment with your spine. (See Figure 9-8, page 82.) Inhale through your nostrils and focus your energy inward.

2. Arch your back up into the Cat Posture, pressing your abdominal muscles into the spine. Drop your neck and head forward, allowing the weight of your head to gently stretch the neck, upper back, and shoulders. (See Figure 9-9, page 82.) Breathe deeply into your chest through your nostrils for a count of 3 breaths.

3. Now release your back, pressing the spine down, reversing the arch of your back into the Dog Posture. Lift your head up while lifting and opening your buttocks. (See Figure 9-10, page 82.) Breathe into this stretch for a count of 3 breaths. Consciously press your hands into the floor and feel a stretch in your upper back and shoulders.

4. Alternate between the Cat and Dog postures 3 times, coming back down into the Table position as your final resting position. Pause for a moment.

### Counter Posture

Come down into the Child Pose. (See Figures 10-1 and 10-2, page 89.)

*continued*

**Figure 9-8**
*Your back and spine are completely flat in the Table position.*

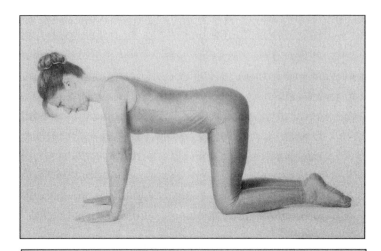

**Figure 9-9**
*Press your abdominal muscles into the spine and drop your neck and head forward into the Cat. Feel the stretch along the spine, upper back, and shoulders.*

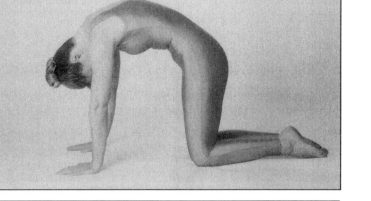

**Figure 9-10**
*Release your back, pressing the spine down, reversing the arch of your back into the Dog. You are feeling a different stretch along your spine and in your upper back area now.*

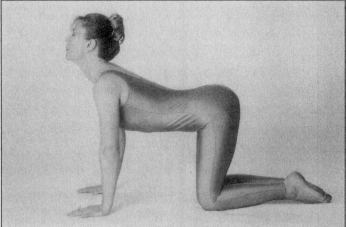

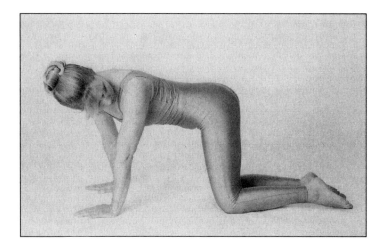

**Figure 9-11**

*As you turn to look at your tailbone, you create a stretch along the opposite side of the body. Keep your arms straight and your spine in alignment with your neck for a proper stretch.*

## Threading the Needle

This is a posture that best follows the Cat and Dog. You twist your body to look behind, creating a deeper stretch in the spine. Feel the stretch along the side of your body and your hip and waist area, as you turn and twist your spine in this stretch.

1. Come into the Table position. Turn your upper body to the left as you try to look at your tailbone. (See Figure 9-11.) Breathe into this stretch for 5 breaths.

2. Bring your body back to the Table position and pause for a moment while breathing in. Close your eyes.

3. Repeat this sequence on the right side.

### *Counter Posture*

Come down into the Child Pose. (See Figures 10-1 and 10-2, page 89.)

## Inverted Dog Posture (*Adho Mukha Svanasana*)

**Focus**

*Bend your knees as much as you need to in order to place your heels into the floor. Work toward straightening your legs, always keeping your knees in a slightly unlocked position.*

This is an energizing posture and a good one to fit into your daily yoga routine. It releases tension in the upper back and behind your shoulder blades. You feel a stretch all over your body: the back of your calves and upper thighs as you press your heels down, and the back of your arms as you press your hands into the floor. You feel a stretch along the back of the neck as your head naturally pulls down on those muscles. You also feel a deep stretch in the upper back and along the entire length of your spine as you drop the shoulder blades into your chest. The Inverted Dog is very beneficial for those suffering from any form of arthritis.

1. Come into the Table position. Tuck your toes under and allow your head and neck to drop forward. (See Figure 9-12.)

2. Lift your body into an inverted "V," adjusting your feet so that they are a little wider than shoulder width apart. Imagine lifting your buttocks square into the ceiling. Allow your head and neck to relax while dropping your shoulders into your chest. Press your buttocks into the ceiling. Fingers are spread apart, middle finger pointing straight ahead. You are looking at your feet. Press your heels down as far as is comfortable. (See Figure 9-13.)

3. Breathe deeply into your chest for 5 breaths. Press your hands into the floor. Feel this stretch energizing your body.

### Counter Posture

Come out of this posture by sliding your feet together, bending the knees forward, and kneeling on the floor. Go into the Child Pose (see Figures 10-1 and 10-2, page 89).

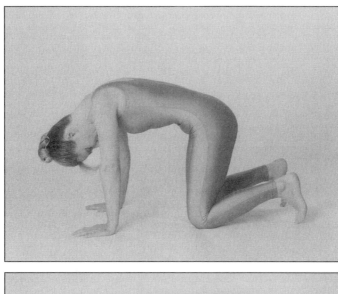

**Figure 9-12**

*Tuck your toes under and drop your head and neck down.*

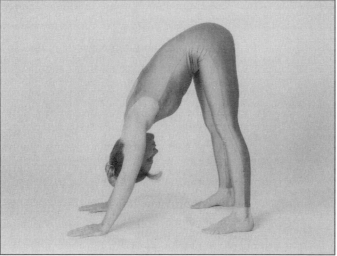

**Figure 9-13**

*Feel the stretch created in your hips and along the length of your legs, into your heels. Drop your shoulders into your chest. Feel the stretch along your spine and upper back and into your arms.*

## Chapter 10

# Counter Postures

In yoga we are always aware of protecting the spine against injury, especially the lower back and neck. With this in mind, there are a series of simple counter postures designed to "counter" any stress placed on the spine during a posture. They help these areas rest and recover after being worked.

Throughout the postures, I always recommend a counter posture to use after any posture that may have been too strenuous. Go into the counter posture directly following the posture, and hold it until you feel you are ready to move on.

Please note that although there may not be a photo of each counter posture when mentioned, it is important to do the counter posture suggested to eliminate any strain placed on the neck and/or back.

## Child Pose (*Darnikasana*)

Reminiscent of the position you were in inside the womb, the Child Pose is the most popular counter posture as it gently and naturally relaxes the spine. As you breathe in and out through your nose, imagine sending your breath to the inside of your lower back. The breath warms and massages you there. To end, place your hands on your lower back if you wish. Feel their warmth. Use the healing energy that is released from your hands as you touch yourself.

1. Come into a kneeling position. Lower your upper body and forehead down onto the floor. Completely relax your shoulders, neck, and face. Rest your arms and hands at your sides. Breathe deeply into your abdomen. (See Figure 10-1.)

2. Extend your arms out in front of you, palms on the floor. Feel the stretch in your upper back. (See Figure 10-2.) Hold this position for as long as you feel necessary.

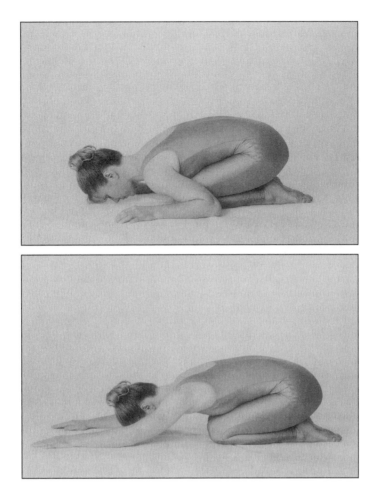

**Figure 10-1**
*Lower your upper body down to the floor. Completely relax.*

**Figure 10-2**
*Feel the stretch in your upper back as you extend your arms out in front of you.*

## Knee to Chest Posture

**Note**

*This posture is also demonstrated in the "Limbering Up" postures in chapter 8.*

Use this as a counter posture whenever you feel the need to release your lower back after a strenuous posture.

1. Come into a lying position with your legs extended. Bend your right knee into your chest and gently press it down. Consciously relax your neck and shoulders and continue breathing through your nostrils. (See Figure 8-1, page 61.)

2. Press your lower back into the floor as you continue to press your knee into your abdomen. Hold for 5 breaths, limbering up the hip area.

3. Slide your right leg down next to your left leg and shake both legs out.

4. Repeat the same sequence with your left leg.

5. Now press both knees into your chest and continue inhaling through your nose. (See Figure 8-2, page 61.)

6. With your arms at your side, rotate your body from side to side, massaging the lower back. Keep both shoulders on the floor and relax your upper body. (See Figure 8-3, page 61.)

7. Slide both legs down back into the lying position. Rest a moment while breathing through your nose.

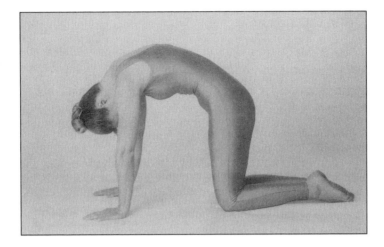

**Figure 10-3**

*Press your abdominal muscles into the spine and drop your neck and head forward into the Cat. Feel the stretch along the spine, upper back, and shoulders.*

## Cat Posture

Use the Cat as a counter posture whenever you need an increased stretch along your entire spine or to allow for a further release in the lower back.

> ### Note
> *This posture is also demonstrated in the "Stretching the Spine" postures in chapter 9.*

1. Come into the Table position. Place your hands and knees shoulder width apart. Arch your back up into the Cat Posture, pressing your abdominal muscles into the spine. (See Figure 10-3.) Allow the neck and head to relax, allowing their weight to gently stretch the neck, upper back, and shoulders. Breathe deeply into your chest for a count of 3 breaths.

2. Release your back and bring yourself down into the Child Pose. (See Figures 10-1 and 10-2, page 89.)

## Lying Spinal Release

This stretch offers a wonderful release for your lower back. Stay in this position until you no longer feel any strain in your lower back, remembering to use your breath to relax these muscles.

1. Come into a tummy position. Extend your arms straight out at your sides. Turn your head to the left, placing your right ear on the floor. (See Figure 10-4.)

2. Lift and swing your left leg up and back over your right hip/buttock area as far as is comfortable. (See Figure 10-5.) Breathe into the stretch for 5 breaths. Use your arms and stationary leg as support.

3. Swing your leg back down. Repeat on the other side, placing your left ear on the floor and swinging your right leg up and over.

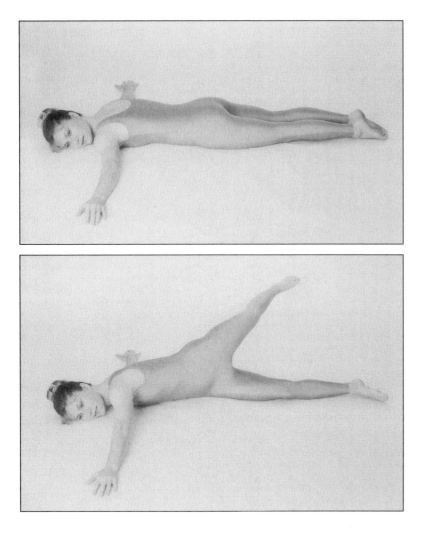

**Figure 10-4**

*Lie on your tummy and turn your head to the left, with your right ear on the floor.*

**Figure 10-5**

*Swing your left leg up and back over your right leg. Keep both arms down to create a twist and gentle release in your lower back.*

## Chapter 11

# Sun Salutation

The Sun Salutation, meaning "salute or greeting to the sun," is an invigorating flow of postures designed to completely work your entire body as it energizes and helps prepare it for further postures. Traditionally, the Sun Salutation was performed before sunrise, which is where it gets its name. Today, it is often performed at the beginning of a yoga session, however, I find it equally pleasing and soothing when done at the end.

If you are a novice to the Sun Salutation, start out slow, taking as many breaths as you need in order to perfect the flow and achieve maximum benefit.

Once you feel you have mastered each posture—and this could take weeks—proceed to the next level. The pace is quickened, coordinating each posture with an inhaling breath, not pausing before smoothly flowing into the next posture with the following exhaling breath, linking your breathing pattern to your body movement.

This can be difficult to master, but the rewards far exceed the work involved. The fluid movement of the postures tone and strengthen your body, encourage deep breathing, and increase blood flow throughout your body.

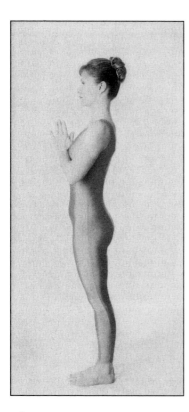

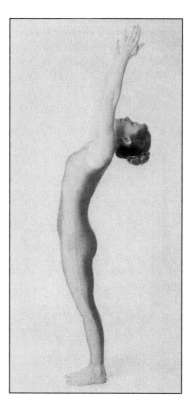

**Figure 11-1**

*Know that as you acknowledge
the external sun, you are also
acknowledging your internal sun.*

**Figure 11-2**

*Imagine picking up the sun
behind you, slightly arching back.
Feel sun's warmth filling you.*

## Sun Salutation (*Surya Namaskar*)

1. Come into a standing position with your feet together. Your hands are together in the prayer position over your heart. Breathe in and out through your nostrils. (See Figure 11-1.)

2. Inhale and raise your arms over your head, keeping them as straight as possible. You are reaching up toward a higher consciousness. Lower your head back while bending your knees slightly. (See Figure 11-2.)

*continued*

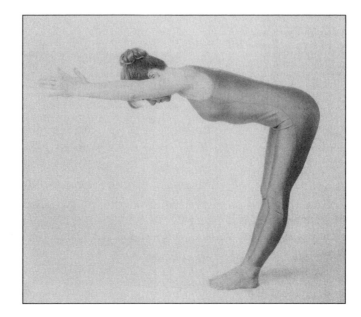

**Figure 11-3**

*Imagine the sun between your hands and feel the warmth of the sun's energy.*

3. Exhale and bring your upper body forward from your hips and stop halfway. Feel the warmth of the sun's energy between your hands. Hold this position for a few breaths and stay connected. (See Figure 11-3.)

4. Continue to lower your upper body until the palms of your hands touch the floor beside your feet, finger-tips even with your toes. Bend your knees as much as is needed in order for you to touch the floor. Relax your head, neck, and shoulders. (See Figure 11-4.)

5. Inhale and stretch your right leg back, keeping your back and extended leg as straight as possible. Allow your right knee to touch the floor, if necessary. Look straight ahead. Feel the stretch. Try and keep your hands in the same position. (See Figure 11-5.)

*continued*

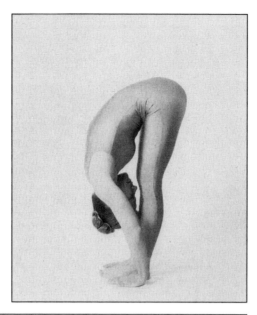

**Figure 11-4**
*Bring the energy down, placing the sun into the ground.*

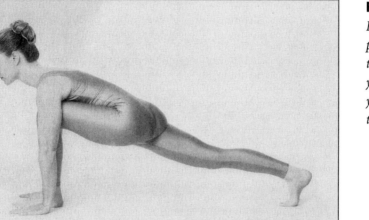

**Figure 11-5**
*Feel the energy in your palms and arms. Use this energy to energize your entire body as you stretch out into the Runner's Stretch.*

**Figure 11-6**
*Hold your breath,
pausing to teach you
to pause in life.*

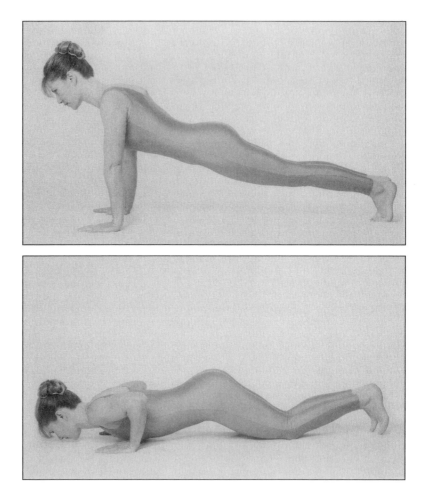

**Figure 11-7**
*Lower your body and
face down in the
respect to the earth.*

6.  Extend your left leg next to your right leg, as if in a
    push-up position. Straighten both legs as you come
    up on your toes. Your arms are straight, supporting
    your body. Try to get your body to form a straight
    line. Hold this position while you hold your breath.
    (See Figure 11-6.)

7.  Exhale and lower your knees, chest, and chin to the
    floor, while bending your elbows. Do not move your
    hands. Lift your buttocks up in the air. (See Figure
    11-7.)

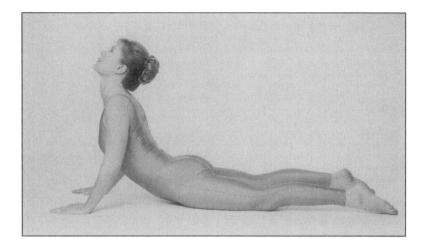

**Figure 11-8**
*Lift your face to the sun. Bring in the energy and see the picture of the sun, the sun's rays glowing out to your Third Eye (forehead).*

8. Inhale and lower your abdomen to the floor. Press your hands into the floor, lifting your upper body. Squeeze your buttocks. Lift your head and gently arch your back as you lower your head back. Your hips and thighs are on the floor. Your chest is open. (See Figure 11-8.) The energy is now moving from your lower back all the way up to your forehead. This is the Cobra position.

**Note**
*The Cobra is described in the Chakra Four postures, chapter 15.*

*continued*

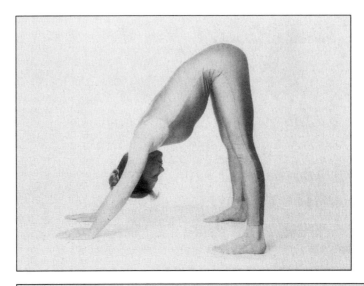

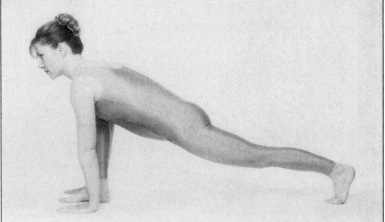

9. Exhale as you tuck your toes under and swing your buttocks up into the Inverted Dog Posture. Allow your head to drop down between your shoulders, dropping your shoulders into your chest. Straighten your arms and legs as much as possible, pressing your heels into the floor. Press your buttocks into the ceiling. (See Figure 11-9.)

10. Inhale and place your right foot between your hands. Stretch your left leg back, keeping your back and extended leg as straight as possible. This is called the

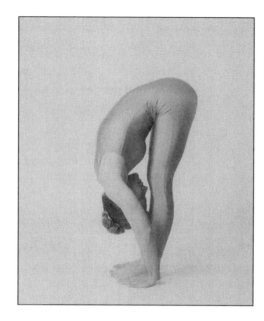

**Figure 11-11**
*Pick the sun up from the ground.*

Runner's Stretch. (See Figure 11-10.) Allow your left knee to touch the floor if necessary. Look straight ahead. Try and keep your hands in the same position.

11. Exhale and bring your left leg forward, placing it next to your right foot. Your hands remain in the same position as you press the palms of your hands into the floor. Bend your knees as much as is needed as you relax your head, neck, and shoulders. (See Figure 11-11.)

*continued*

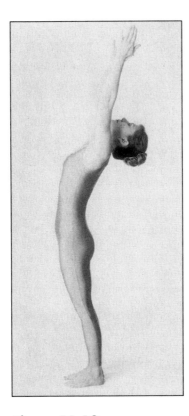

**Figure 11-12**

*Lift up the sun as you bring your arms up over your head. Look up and place the sun back into the sky above you.*

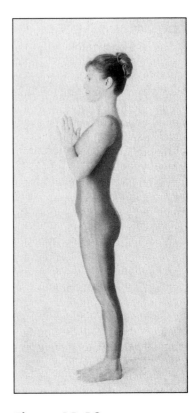

**Figure 11-13**

*Feel the peace inside you and the activation of your Heart center.*

12. Inhale and slowly stretch up, keeping them as straight as possible. Lower your head back as far as is comfortable, arching slightly. (See Figure 11-12.)

13. Exhale as you lower your arms, palms together, back into the prayer position over your heart. (See Figure 11-13.)

14. Lower your arms down to the side of your body. Rest for a few breaths.

15. Repeat steps 1–14 with your left leg.

Chapter 12

# Chakra One Postures

The first chakra deals with your relationship to yourself. As you strengthen it through postures, you help yourself become grounded and more comfortable with yourself. It is here that you begin to break away from societal beliefs, feeling strong and secure in your own beliefs and with who you are.

The following brief meditation is to help activate the energy of your first chakra. Your focus goes inward as you become aware of the body parts involved in this chakra, as well as the emotional meaning attached to it.

The chakra continues to open and balance as you engage in the postures that correspond to your first chakra's body parts. The postures for the first energy center are designed to send energy to the lower part of your body.

*Focus your attention to the very base of your spine, your tailbone, where you see the color ruby red. Visualize a band of ruby red in the front and behind your tailbone as you breathe in the energy of the ruby red. Feel the energy. Work with this energy as it anchors you into the ground, anchoring your energy to Mother Earth. Know you are fully anchored.*

*Make a commitment to be here in your physical body—fully. Now that you are firmly rooted to Earth, you feel safe and secure, fully grounded and nurtured by the energy of Mother Earth. Look to your first energy center and see it radiating the color ruby red.*

*As you breathe in the ruby red, affirm to yourself:*

*"I am safe and secure."*

*Activate the vibration of the color so that you can start to feel the quality of the affirmation.*

Now that you're in your first energy center, let's begin to strengthen it.

## Staff Pose (*Dandasana*)

The Staff Pose helps encourage the straightening of the spine, preparing it for any seated postures and twists. It particularly creates the proper body alignment in which to perform the seated forward bends in this chapter, sending the message to the body to maintain proper posture in order to protect it and achieve the most benefit from the postures.

Feel the chest opening and the spine stretching as you sit up completely straight. You feel a stretch in your shoulders and arms as you press your hands into the floor. Your spine is straightened. Your thighs are strengthened and your hamstrings, calves, and heels are stretched as you flex your toes.

1. Come into a sitting position with your legs extended and feet together. Focus your attention on your spine, on your posture. Adjust your buttocks so that you are sitting comfortably on both sitting bones with your spine straight.

2. Place the palms of your hands on the floor next to your buttocks. Press them into the floor with your fingers facing forward. As you press your hands into the floor, feel the spine straightening. Imagine a string attached to your Crown chakra, the top of your head, and imagine someone pulling on this string to help straighten the spine further. You are sending a message to your body as to what it feels like to properly sit up straight, to have good body alignment with the spine straight and the head resting comfortably above the spine.

*continued*

**Figure 12-1**

*The Staff Pose is a preparatory pose, properly aligning your body before moving into more intense seated bends.*

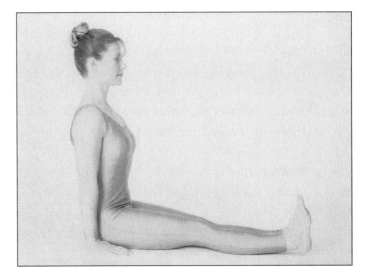

3. Squeeze your abdominal muscles into the spine to help keep the spine straight as you consciously relax your upper body. Tense your thigh muscles as you flex your toes, pulling them back toward you. (See Figure 12-1.) Focus on your posture. Breathe into your chest for a count of 5 breaths.

4. You are now ready to proceed safely into the Seated Forward Bend Series that follows. Stay focused on your spine. Remember that this is what it feels like to hold your spine straight and erect.

# Seated Forward Bend Series
## (*Upavista Konasanas*)

The Seated Forward Bend Series is a series of three postures designed to stretch your lower body. The series is composed of the following postures: Open Leg Forward Bend, Open Leg Center Forward Bend, and Closed Leg Forward Bend. They are listed on pages 110–115.

Keeping your abdominal muscles pulled into your spine will allow you to pull your upper body down more easily. Feel the energy being pushed into the lower part of your body—your first energy center—as you bend forward into these postures. Feel your mind become quiet.

Go slowly through this series, listening to your body. Do not push yourself into any of these stretches. Your muscles have a memory and they will become more flexible. As you breathe into the stretches, you'll feel your muscles begin to relax, allowing you to go further into the stretch.

Remember to always keep your knees in an unlocked position throughout this series, never fully straightening them. This protects them from overextension.

### Focus
*Throughout this series, always keep your knees in an unlocked position to protect them, never fully straightening or overextending them.*

# Open Leg Forward Bend (*Parsva Upavista Konasana*)

This first posture in the series can be done with both legs open or with one leg tucked into your groin, whichever is most comfortable for you.

1. Come into the Staff Pose. (See Figure 12-1, page 108.) Open your legs, stretching them out as far as is comfortable. Focus on your spine, keeping it straight and erect. (See Figure 12-2.)

2. Turn your upper body to the right and place your hands on the floor, on either side of your right knee. Exhale as you lower your upper body over your right leg. (See Figure 12-3.) Your knees stay in a slightly unlocked position. Your spine is straight with your head and neck in alignment. Breathe into the stretch for 5 breaths, pressing your hands into the floor and relaxing your upper body. Both sitting bones remain on the floor.

3. Come back up to center and pause for a few breaths. Repeat this sequence with your left leg.

4. Come back up to center and slide the legs together, stretched out in front of you. Gently shake both legs out while you pause for a few breaths.

## Variation

In step 1, bend one leg in, tucking your foot into your groin, if opening both legs is difficult or causes too much strain. Continue on with remaining steps. (See Figure 12-4.)

Remember to press your abdominal muscles into your spine to help straighten the spine. This helps you to lower the body down further, but only going as far as your comfort level permits. You are not lowering your upper body by using your head. Focus on your abdominal muscles to help pull your body down. This is a first chakra posture, so you are engaging your lower body to pull the upper body down. You should not feel any strain in the upper body.

## Comfort Aid

*If performing the posture with one leg bent in and you still feel tightness in your knee when lowering your body over the extended leg, support your bent knee with a folded towel or blanket.*

*If your sitting bone lifts off the floor when lowering your body, sit on a folded towel or blanket.*

*If your hamstrings are tight and you are having difficulty lowering your upper body, wrap a belt or towel around your foot on the extended leg and pull on the towel to help lower your upper body.*

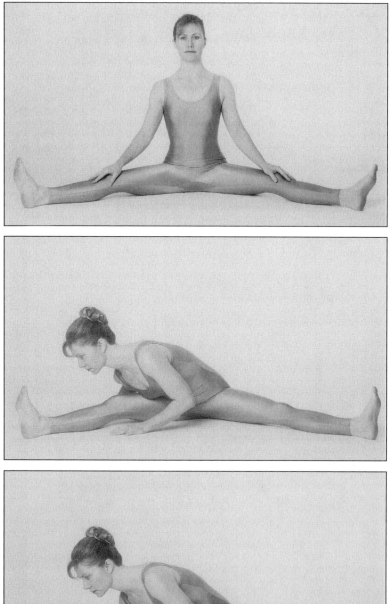

**Figure 12-2**

*Focus on your spine. You are comfortably sitting as straight as you can, your abdominal muscles pulled in to support your spine.*

**Figure 12-3**

*Remember to lead with your chest, keeping your shoulders as level as possible.*

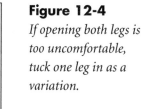

**Figure 12-4**

*If opening both legs is too uncomfortable, tuck one leg in as a variation.*

## Open Leg Center Forward Bend
## (*Upavista Konasana*)

1. Coming from the Staff Pose (Figure 12-1, page 108) or Open Leg Forward Bend (page 110), open your legs once again, stretching them out as far as is comfortable. Focus on your spine, keeping it straight and erect. Place the palms of your hands on the floor in front of you. (See Figure 12-5.)

2. Exhale and "walk" your hands down, lowering your upper body by using your abdominal muscles. Lead with your chest, keeping your shoulders as level as possible. Your neck is in alignment with your spine. Go only as far as your comfort level permits. Look straight ahead. (See Figure 12-6.)

3. Now flex your toes and hold this position for 3 breaths. Relax the toes and hold this position for another 3 breaths.

4. Walk your hands back up to center. Slide your legs together and shake them out.

### Advanced

Coming from step 2, keep walking your hands down, bringing your chest down to the floor. You are pulling your upper body down by squeezing your abdominal muscles. Grab hold of your ankles or feet. As you exhale, bring your chest down as close to the floor as is comfortable. Your neck and upper back are relaxed enough to look straight ahead. (See Figure 12-7.) Breathe into the stretch in the back of your legs for 5 breaths.

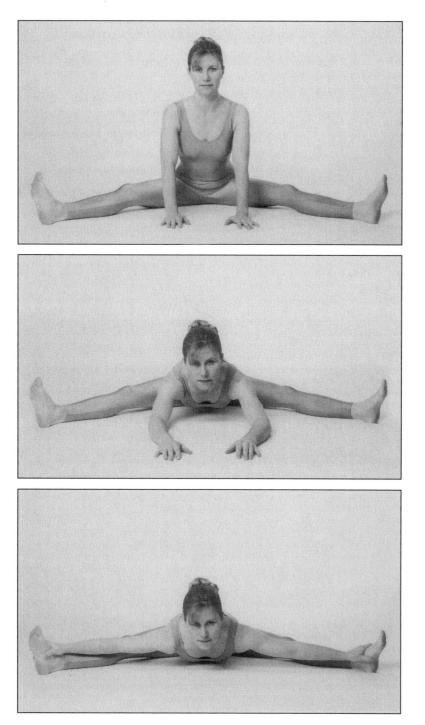

**Figure 12-5**
*Place your hands on the floor in front of you.*

**Figure 12-6**
*Walk your hands down, lowering yourself using your abdominal muscles, bending at the hips. There should be no strain in your upper body.*

**Figure 12-7**
*Feel the difference as you lower your chest to the floor. Your upper body is now engaged, adding a stretch to the entire length of your spine.*

# Closed Leg Forward Bend (*Pascimottanasana*)

This is the last posture in the Seated Forward Bend Series.

### Comfort Aid

*If you cannot reach your ankles or your toes, flex your feet to feel an added stretch.*

*If your hamstrings are tight and you are having difficulty lowering your upper body over the extended leg, wrap a belt or towel around your feet and pull on the towel.*

*If your hips are tight, sit on a folded towel or blanket when lowering your upper body.*

*To help eliminate any strain on your back when ending the posture, place a folded towel or blanket on your shins to rest your forehead on.*

1. Come into a sitting position with your legs extended. Exhale and lower your upper body over your legs. Relax your upper body, neck, and shoulders as you lower, using your abdominal muscles and leading with your chest. Your head is in alignment with your spine. Breathe into the stretch for 3 breaths. Grab hold of your ankles, keeping your spine completely straight. Hold this position for 3 breaths. (See Figure 12-8.)

2. Now grab hold of your toes, if you can, and pull the toes toward you to enhance the stretch in the back of the calves and heels. (See Figure 12-9.) Breathe into this stretch for 3 breaths.

3. Release and shake the legs out.

4. To end, relax your neck and lower your forehead down to your knees. Grab hold of your feet or ankles. (See Figure 12-10.) Feel the difference in the stretch. You are now engaging your upper body as you feel a nice stretch in your lower back and all the way up your spine, as well as the back of the legs.

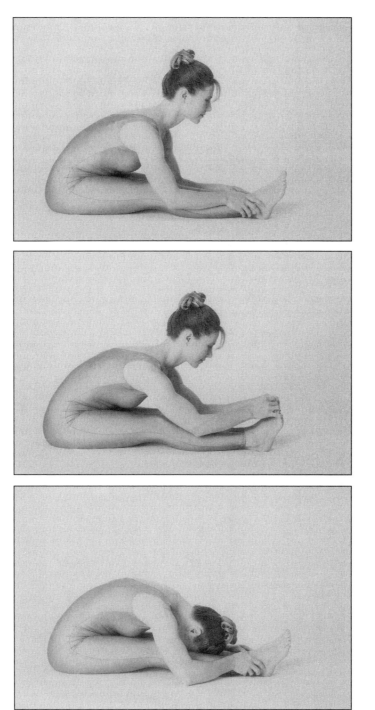

**Figure 12-8**

*Lower your upper body, leading with your chest, and grab hold of your ankles.*

**Figure 12-9**

*Enhance the stretch by grabbing your toes.*

**Figure 12-10**

*Lower your forehead to your knees, feeling a stretch all the way up the spine and back of the legs.*

# Runner's Stretch

This is wonderful for stretching the back of the legs, arms, upper thighs, groin, and hip area. Feel the energy being pushed down as you press your palms into the floor.

1.  Come into the Table position. Bring your right foot forward between your hands. Your toes should be as even as possible with your fingertips. Extend your left leg behind you, supporting this leg on your toes. (See Figure 12-11.) Continue to press your hands into the floor, keeping your back straight and your head in alignment with your spine. Try to create a straight line with your body. Hold this position for 5 breaths.

2.  To come out of the posture safely, lower your left knee down to the floor. (See Figure 12-12.)

3.  Sit back onto your left foot, extending your right leg out. Lower your upper body over your right leg by squeezing your abdominal muscles into your spine. Your head is in alignment with your spine. (See Figure 12-13.)

4.  Come back into the Table position and rest for a few breaths.

5.  Repeat this sequence, switching the legs.

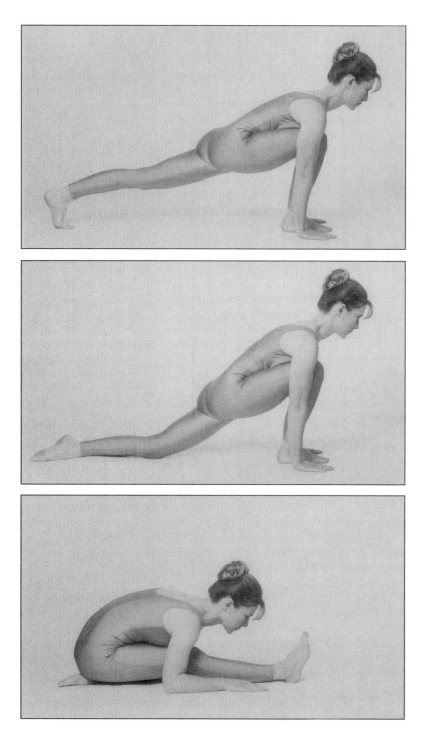

**Figure 12-11**

*Imagine creating a diagonal line with your body. Feel the energy being pushed down as you press your palms into the floor.*

**Figure 12-12**

*To safely come out of this, lower your left knee down to the floor.*

**Figure 12-13**

*As a reverse stretch, lower your body over the extended leg. Feel the stretch in the hamstring.*

## Leg Raises (*Urdhva Prasarita Padasana*)

Whenever you don't feel grounded, your energy isn't flowing through your first chakra body parts. Doing this posture will help you to focus on your first energy center and help you feel grounded, completely safe and secure. When you inhale, send the oxygen—the energy—to your first energy center at the base of the spine. Stay focused on what is happening to your body during this posture. Know that energy blocks are being released as you exhale.

You are engaging your lower body in this posture, so from the waist up, set the intention to relax your upper body—and it will. Synchronize your breathing with the leg movements, inhaling as you lift your leg, exhaling as you lower it.

1. Come into a lying position with your knees bent. Extend your left leg out. Your arms are at your sides. Relax your upper body. (See Figure 12-14.)

2. Squeeze your buttocks and press your lower back into the floor. Inhale, flex your foot, and slowly lift your left leg as high as is comfortable. Keep your leg as straight as you can. When you reach your comfort level, press your foot into the ceiling for 3 breaths. (See Figure 12-15.)

3. Now point your foot as you breathe for 5 breaths. Feel the part of the body being activated.

4. Begin to slowly lower the leg to the floor, keeping your foot pointed. Press your lower back and right foot into the floor to protect your lower back. (See Figure 12-16.)

5. Lower your leg to a point 1–2 inches above the floor and hold. (See Figure 12-17, page 120.) Pause for a few breaths, squeezing your buttocks, and staying in your first energy center. Stay grounded. Do not touch the floor.

6. Repeat steps 2–4 two more times. On your second lift, once you reach as high as is comfortable, point and flex your foot for 3 breaths. On your third lift, do ankle circles for 3 breaths. Try not to touch the floor until all three sets are completed.

*continued*

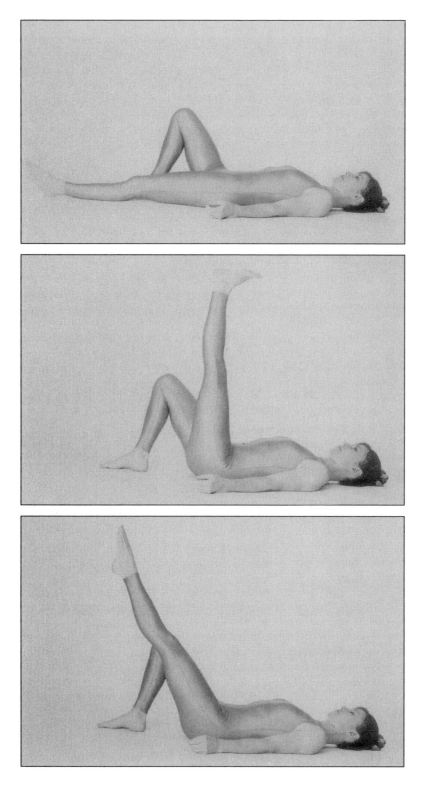

**Figure 12-14**
*Extend your left leg out as you relax your upper body.*

**Figure 12-15**
*Inhale, flex your foot, and slowly lift your left leg as high as is comfortable, squeezing your buttocks to protect your lower back.*

**Figure 12-16**
*Begin to lower your leg, pressing your lower back and foot into the floor once again for support.*

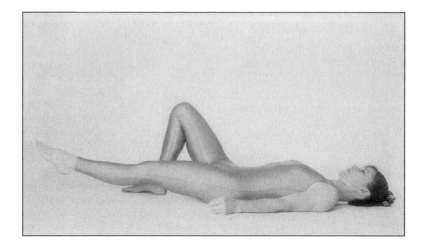

**Figure 12-17**
*Lower your leg to a point 1–2 inches above the floor and hold. Remember to breathe as you hold the posture.*

7. Bring the left leg down to a resting position, sliding the right leg down to meet the left. Shake the legs out. Feel the difference between the legs. Feel the energy running through the left leg. It feels lighter and longer.

8. Now balance the body by repeating the sequence with the right leg. Close your eyes so you feel what's happening.

## Counter Posture

Press your knees into your chest. Rotate your knees from side to side, gently massaging the lower back as you do so. Both shoulders remain on the floor.

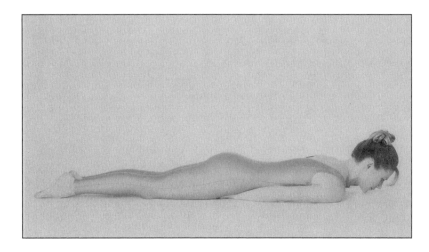

**Figure 12-18**

*Bring your head forward so that your nose and chin are lightly brushing the floor. Your fist under your groin serves to protect your spine.*

## Locust (*Salabhasana*)

You get into the Locust position by turning over onto your tummy (abdomen). Make the transition without disrupting the energy in your body. Integrate this flow into your body—the flow of gently moving into another position by disrupting the least amount of energy as possible. You then learn to bring this into your daily life, moving from one task to another with ease and focus.

Focus on where the energy is throughout this posture. Keep your nose and chin down as you lift your legs because you want the energy to stay down. Feel the energy in the back of your legs and lower back when in the full extension of this posture. This posture will help strengthen a weak lower back.

*Note:* Do not do this posture if you are pregnant.

1. Come into a tummy position. Place your palms on the floor, shoulder width apart. Make a fist with your right hand and place it underneath your right groin area. Bring your head forward so that your nose and chin are lightly brushing the floor. (See Figure 12-18.)

*continued*

### Focus

*Keep your leg as straight as you can when lifting it up. As soon as you feel the need to bend your leg, you've gone far enough. It is more important to keep your leg straight than it is to get it up high. Gradually work toward lifting your leg up higher.*

2. Inhale, squeeze your buttocks, and lift your right leg as you point your toe. (See Figure 12-19.) The tighter you squeeze your buttocks, the higher you will be able to lift your leg. If you feel a strain in the lower back you are lifting too high. Lower your leg a little. Completely relax your upper body.

3. Exhale and lower your leg down. Place your head to one side to relax the neck. Remove your hand from your groin and place it back on the floor, shoulder width apart. Rest for a few breaths.

4. Repeat steps 2 and 3 with your left leg.

5. Place both fists under your groin area and lift both legs at the same time. (See Figure 12-20.) Remember to squeeze your buttocks to protect your lower back while you lift. Relax your neck and upper body. Do not rest your face on the floor.

## Variation

This variation works the same muscles, your legs and lower back, as well as works to strengthen a weak lower back. It is simply a safe variation to the Locust, adding interest to your yoga program. This variation is also a good alternative to the Locust when you are pregnant.

In step 1, come into the Table position instead. Squeeze your buttocks and lift your right leg up behind you. Point your toe. Keep your head in alignment to your spine. Keep your leg as straight as you can. (See Figure 12-21.) Lower your leg and rest a few breaths. Repeat with your left leg.

## Counter Posture

Go into the Child Pose (see Figures 10-1 and 10-2, page 89) and then further into the Cat Posture (see Figure 10-3, page 91), if necessary, to release your lower back.

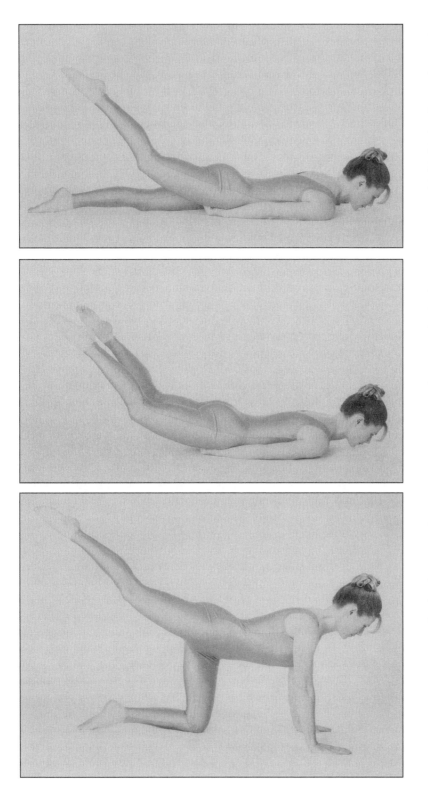

**Figure 12-19**
*The tighter you squeeze your buttocks, the higher you will be able to lift your leg. If you feel any strain in your lower back, lower your leg and tighten your buttocks.*

**Figure 12-20**
*Lift both legs at the same time, again squeezing your buttocks. Focus on where you feel the stretch—your lower back. Remember to breathe.*

**Figure 12-21**
*As a variation, start in the Table position and then lift your leg. Remember to squeeze your buttocks to protect your lower back.*

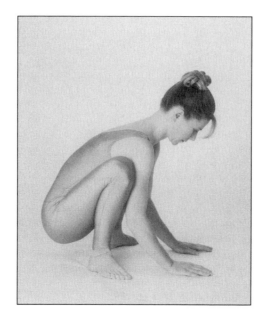

## Elephant Posture (*Uttanasana*)

The Elephant Posture is used to get into a standing position, or to come down into a sitting position. Imagine your arms and head as an extension of an elephant's trunk as you roll your spine up or down, feeling their weight gently stretching your neck and upper back. Feel a nice stretch along the back of your arms and legs as you press the palms of your hands into the floor. Push the energy right down to the soles of your feet, sending it down to Mother Earth.

*Note:* The squatting position is an especially good stretch if you are pregnant, as long as you take it slow and easy.

### Seated to Standing Position

1. Come into a squat position. Position your feet to allow room for your arms inside of your knees. Place the palms of your hands on the floor in front of you. (See Figure 12-22.)

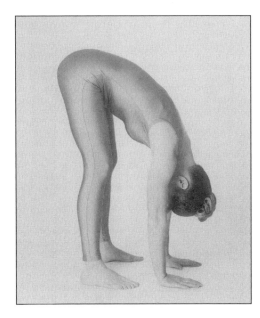

**Figure 12-23**

*Feel a stretch along the back of your arms and legs as you press your hands into the floor.*

2.  Transfer your weight onto your hands, lifting your buttocks up. Bend your knees slightly to protect your lower back and knees, keeping your legs as straight as you can. Allow your head, neck, and shoulders to completely relax. Begin breathing through your nostrils. (See Figure 12-23.)

3.  Press the palms of your hands into the floor and hold for 5 breaths, pushing the energy right down to the soles of the feet. This is a first energy posture, so you are keeping the energy to the lower part of the body.

4.  Inhale and begin slowly raising your upper body, vertebra by vertebra. Your knees remain slightly bent. Pause halfway. Completely relax your upper body and allow the head to drop down between your shoulders. (See Figure 12-24, page 126.)

*continued*

### Focus
*Bend your knees as much as necessary to comfortably place your hands on the floor.*

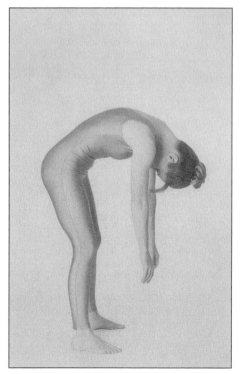

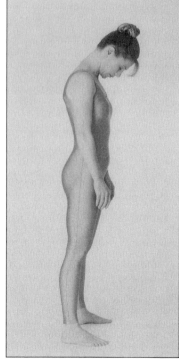

**Figure 12-24**

*Inhale and begin slowly raising your upper body, vertebra by vertebra. Pause halfway. Feel a gentle stretch in your upper back and neck.*

**Figure 12-25**

*Continue to lift the upper body, your head being last to come up.*

5. Continue to lift the upper body until you come to a full standing position. Your head is the last to come up. Your feet are shoulder width apart. (See Figure 12-25.)

6. Stand and center, with your head up, breathing through your nostrils. (See Figure 12-26.) You are now ready to go into any of the standing postures.

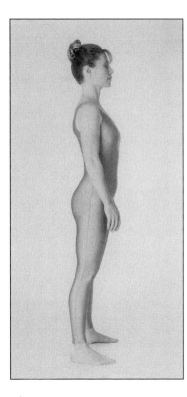

**Figure 12-26**

*Stand and center with your head up.*

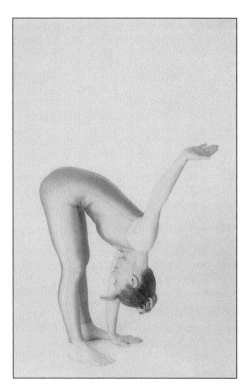

**Figure 12-27**

*As a variation, lift your right arm up for an extra stretch in the shoulders and arms.*

## Variation

1. From step 2, lift your right arm up. Keep your arm straight and hold for 5 breaths. Flex your hand so your palm is flat into the ceiling. (See Figure 12-27.) Feel the extra stretch in the shoulders and arms.

2. Lower your arm and press both palms into the floor.

3. Lift your left arm up.

*continued*

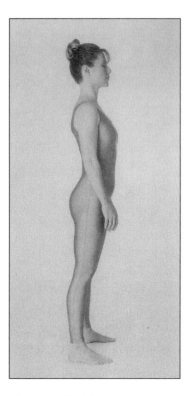

**Figure 12-28**
*Start in the basic standing position.*

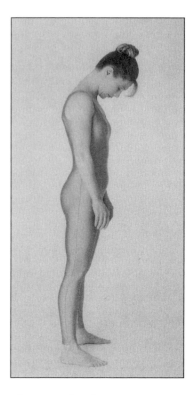

**Figure 12-29**
*Lower your head first.*

## Standing to Seated Position

The Elephant is reversed to come from a standing position into a seated one.

1. Stand and center, breathing through your nostrils. Your eyes are closed. Your feet are shoulder width apart. (See Figure 12-28.)

2. Lower your chin to your chest. (See Figure 12-29.)

3. Inhale and begin slowly lowering your upper body, vertebra by vertebra. Your knees remain slightly bent. Pause halfway. Completely relax your upper body and

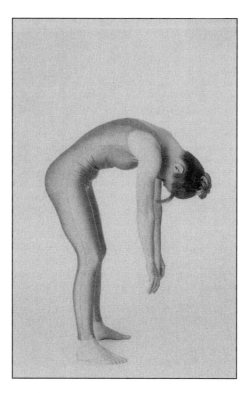

**Figure 12-30**
*Bend your knees as you lower down to protect your spine. Feel the stretch along your spine, upper back, and neck area.*

allow the head to drop down between your shoulders. (See Figure 12-30.)

4.  Lower your upper body all the way down until your hands reach the floor in front of you. Press the palms of your hands into the floor. (See Figure 12-31, page 130.) Bend your knees slightly to protect your lower back and knees, but keeping your legs as straight as you can. Allow your head, neck, and shoulders to completely relax. Begin breathing through your nostrils. Hold for 5 breaths, pushing the energy right down to the soles of the feet. This is a first energy

*continued*

**Figure 12-31**

*Push the energy right down to the soles of the feet.*

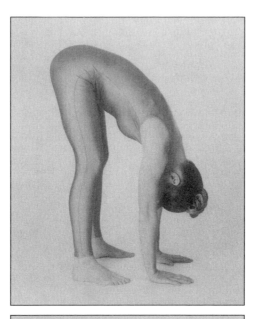

**Figure 12-32**

*Finish in the squat position, coming down into a seated position when ready.*

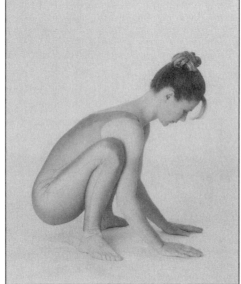

posture so you are keeping the energy to the lower part of the body.

5. Lower your buttocks to come into a squat position. Keeps your hands on the floor in front of you. (See Figure 12-32.)

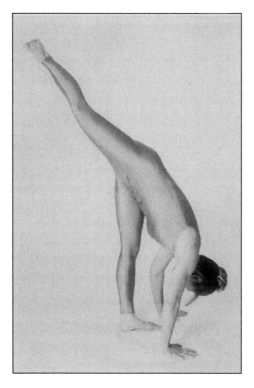

**Figure 12-33**
*Feel your right hip and buttock area being worked as you lift and straighten the leg. Relax your head down.*

## Elephant to Standing Leg Raise (*Uttanasana II*)

This starts out the same as the Elephant Posture, but now you lift one leg back to work and tone your buttocks and hip area, giving the groin area a nice stretch. This is a tough one, but you'll like the lasting results. Keep your leg as straight as you can to lengthen and tone your leg muscles, then work toward lifting it higher.

1.  Come into a squat position. Place the palms of your hands onto the floor in front of you. (See Figure 12-32, page 130.)

*continued*

2. Transfer your weight onto your hands, lifting your buttocks up. Bend your knees slightly to protect your lower back and knees, keeping your legs as straight as you can. Allow your head, neck and shoulders to completely relax. Begin breathing through your nostrils. (See Figure 12-31, page 130.)

3. Squeeze your buttocks and lift your right leg up behind you, keeping it as straight as you can. Flex your foot. (See Figure 12-33, page 131.) Feel your right hip and buttock area being worked. Relax your head down. Lower your chest into your standing leg. Your standing leg remains in a locked position.

4. Lower your right leg and press both palms into the floor as you shake your legs out.

5. Repeat with your left leg.

Chapter 13

# Chakra Two Postures

Bring your focus inward once again as you perform this brief meditation to help activate the energy of your second chakra. You become aware of the body parts involved in this chakra, as well as the emotional meaning. The chakra continues to open and balance as you engage in the postures that correspond to your second chakra's body parts.

*Allow yourself to center for a moment. As you move upward from your first energy center, move your awareness to your lower abdominal area, above your tailbone. You see a beautiful orange. You are in your Creative center. You create with love and use the orange color to do so. It is here that you learn to live in a place of fullness, creating abundance in your life. As you breathe in the orange, draw into your life whatever you need to feel comfortable, and affirm: "I create with love."*

*Your second energy center deals with your relationships with others and how you relate to them on a one-to-one basis. Working on this chakra will help get you in touch with your feelings, your sexuality, your basic sense of acceptance.*

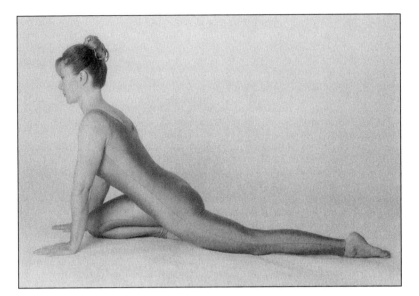

**Figure 13-1**

*Sit on your right foot and properly align your body as you extend your left leg back. Begin to feel a stretch in the upper thigh as the leg is stretched back.*

*Now that you are in your Creative center, begin to strengthen it. Breathe in deeply while you visualize a band of orange in the front and behind your spine. Honor your second energy center. Be calm. Feel the energy. Become a creator with love as you open your second energy center.*

## Extended Leg Pose (*Utthita Eka Padasana*)

Feel the hip socket opening up as you alternately extend your legs back, opening the chest, stretching all the muscles in your upper legs, especially the muscles in your thighs.

1. Come into a kneeling position. Place your hands on the floor in front of you and extend your left leg back. Breathe through your nose as you feel your chest opening up. Feel the body parts being used. (See Figure 13-1.)

2. Bend your left leg and grab hold of your foot with your left hand. Gently press your foot into your buttock. Place your right hand on the floor in front of you. Look ahead. (See Figure 13-2.)

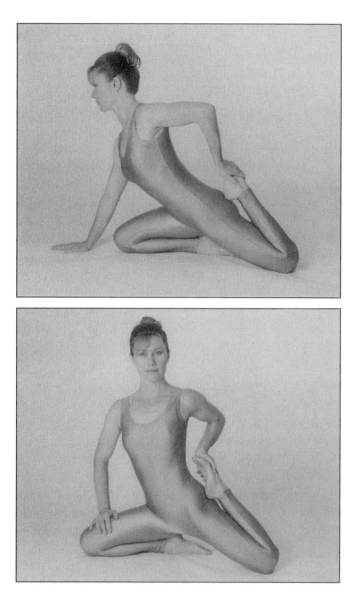

**Figure 13-2**

*Gently press your foot into your buttock. Feel a deep stretch created in your thigh, from your hips all the way down to the top of your knee.*

**Figure 13-3**

*Breathe into the stretch to help relax the muscles engaged.*

3. Turn your upper body to the left so that your hips are facing out and to your left. (See Figure 13-3.) Breathe into the stretch to help relax the muscles engaged. Your right hand is on your right knee, or on the floor in front of you, to help

*continued*

support the upper body. Squeeze your buttocks and your abdominal muscles to help straighten and support your spine. Hold for 5 breaths.

4. Release the left leg, extending it out behind you. Slide your left leg back under your buttocks so you are again in a kneeling position. Pause for a moment.

5. Repeat this sequence with your right leg.

## Counter Posture

Come down into the Child Pose. (See Figures 10-1 and 10-2, page 89.) Rest for 5 breaths.

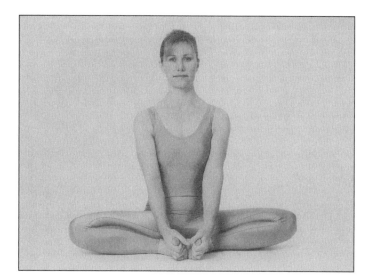

**Figure 13-4**
*Sit up as straight as you can as you gently pull your heels into your groin. Press your knees into the floor once your heels are positioned. Feel the stretch in your groin and inner thighs.*

## Butterfly Pose (*Baddha Konasana*)

This is a calming, gentle posture designed to help release your hip area, stretch your groin muscles, and ease lower back pain. When you lift your knees up and down, as if flapping the wings of a butterfly, you begin to tone your inner thighs. Notice the difference in the ending stretch as you slide your feet forward, away from your groin. Feel new muscles being engaged. You feel a deeper stretch in your hips, lower back, and the backs of your legs.

*Note:* The Butterfly is especially beneficial for pregnant women as it opens the hips to prepare the body for childbirth.

1. Coming from a comfortable seated position, bring the soles of your feet together, sitting up as straight as you can. Grab hold of your toes or ankles and gently pull your feet into your groin, only as far as you comfortably can, without affecting your posture. Sit up straight and feel your chest open.

*continued*

**Comfort Aid**
*If it is difficult for you to sit up comfortably in this position, sit on 2 or 3 towels to lift your hips higher than your knees. This will also make it easier to press your knees down.*

**Figure 13-5**

*Slowly lift the knees up and down to help tone your inner thighs.*

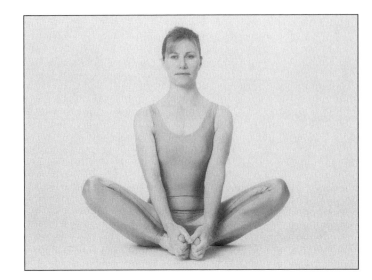

### Focus

*Keep your spine as straight as you can at all times. Press your knees down only as far as they can comfortably go without rounding your back. Take your time.*

2. Press your knees into the floor while breathing into your chest. Press gently without straining the muscles in your inner thigh or groin. Hold this position for 10 breaths. (See Figure 13-4, page 137.)

3. Slowly lift your knees up and down, as if lifting the wings of the butterfly. (See Figure 13-5.)

## Counter Posture

Sit up and shake your legs out.

## Advanced

1. Coming from step 1, exhale and bend your upper body forward from your hips, using your abdominal muscles and leading with your chin. Press your elbows into your knees or thighs, wherever they touch. Place your chest to your feet as close as possible as you look up and extend your upper body

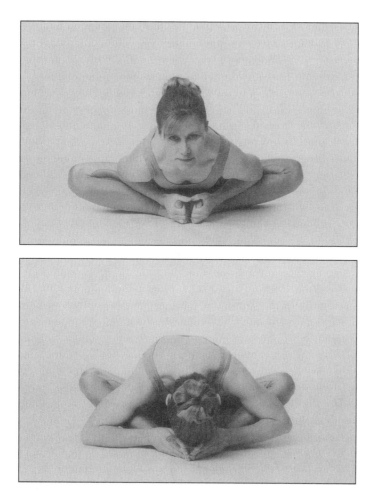

**Figure 13-6**

*Increase the stretch in your groin by lowering your upper body, bending at the hips. Your upper body and neck are relaxed enough to look straight ahead.*

**Figure 13-7**

*Feel a different stretch as you engage the upper body by lowering with your forehead—an added stretch along the spine as well as in the hips.*

forward. (See Figure 13-6.) Relax your shoulders, pushing them down from your ears to prevent hunching. Breathe through your nostrils, holding for 10 breaths.

2. Sit up and slide your feet forward, keeping the soles of your feet touching. Your spine is straight. Pause for a moment.

3. Lower your head as you lower your upper body once again, leading with your forehead. Hold on to your toes as you place your forehead on your feet. (See Figure 13-7.) Notice the difference in the stretch, the different muscles being engaged.

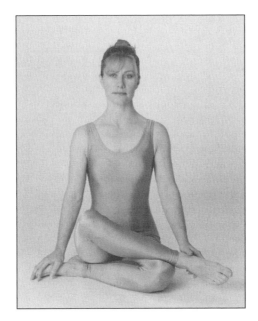

## Hip Tendon Stretch

Although not a traditional yoga posture, the Hip Tendon Stretch is useful as part of your daily program. The tendons and muscles inside your hip socket tend to become tight, and over time, inflexible. It is important to keep them flexible and healthy as it is these muscles that help support the hip joint, protecting the body against injury as you age, such as a broken hip from a fall.

1. Come into a comfortable seated position. Place your right ankle on your left knee, tucking your left leg beside or under your right buttock. (See Figure 13-8.) Focus on your hip tendon, sending your breath to your right hip joint to help relax these muscles. Hold for 5 breaths.

2. Place the palms of your hands on the floor in front of you, relaxing your neck and upper back. Look down at the floor. Hold for 5 breaths, focusing on the deeper stretch in your right hip joint. (See Figure 13-9.)

### Extra Help

*If you cannot place your ankle onto the opposite knee or calf area, place it onto your opposite ankle (crossing the ankles) just as long as one leg is "raised," with one leg on top of the other.*

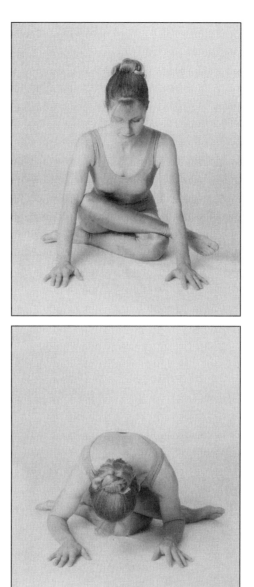

**Figure 13-9**
*Feel a deeper stretch in the second position, remembering to breathe to help relax the muscles engaged.*

**Figure 13-10**
*Go into the third position only if the hip tendon is flexible enough. If it hurts, go back up to the second position.*

3. Lower your upper body further, placing your elbows on the floor ahead of you, relaxing your neck and upper back. (See Figure 13-10.) Be careful not to force the body into this position. Feel a deep stretch in the hip tendon. Breathe into this stretch for 5 breaths.

*continued*

**Figure 13-11**

*For a deeper stretch, place your right knee directly over your left knee. Listen to your body. Don't push yourself into an uncomfortable position.*

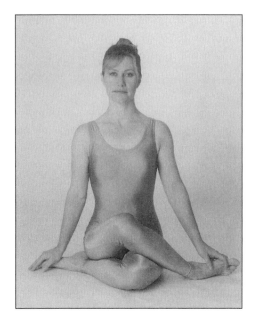

4. Place your soles together and shake out your legs. Straighten both legs and shake them out.

5. Repeat this sequence with the right leg.

## Advanced

As you tuck your left leg under your right buttock in step 1, work toward placing your right knee directly over your left knee to create a deeper stretch. (See Figure 13-11.)

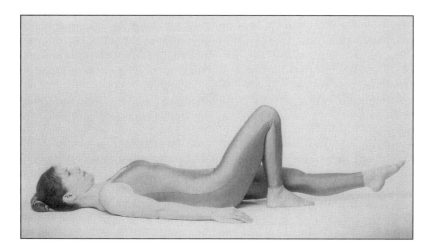

**Figure 13-12**
*Press your lower back
and right foot into the
floor to help support
your spine.*

## Side Leg Raises (*Parsva Urdhva Prasarita Padasana*)

This posture is related to the leg raises performed in Chakra One postures and is an excellent choice for opening the hips while strengthening and toning your upper thighs and buttocks.

Feel the parts of the body engaged as the energy flows there throughout this posture. You are engaging your lower body, so from the waist up, set the intention to relax your upper body, and it will. Synchronize your breath with the leg movement, inhaling as you lift your leg, exhaling as you lower it. If your leg becomes tired, visualize sending your breath to these muscles to help energize them.

Always keep your leg as straight as possible when lifting it. If you feel the need to bend the leg, you have lifted high enough. It is more important to keep the leg straight than it is to get it up higher.

1. Come into a lying position with your knees bent. Extend your left leg out, pointing your foot. Your arms are at the sides of your body. (See Figure 13-12.)

*continued*

**Figure 13-13**

*Feel your hip opening
as you swing your leg
out to the side.*

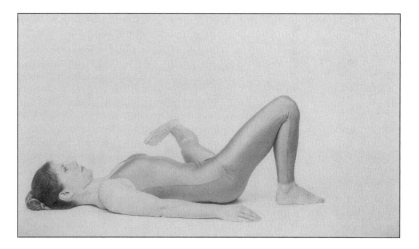

**Focus**

*Remember to
protect the lower
back throughout
this posture by
pressing the
lower back and
the right foot into
the floor, along
with squeezing
the buttocks.*

2. Squeeze your buttocks and press your lower back into the floor. Flex your left foot and swing it out to the left side of your body, keeping it as straight as possible. (See Figure 13-13.) Hold this position for 3 breaths.

3. Inhale and lift the left leg up to center as you press your lower back and right foot into the floor. Lift your left leg up as high as is comfortable, keeping it stretched out and straight as possible. Flex your foot and press it into the ceiling, holding this position for 5 breaths. (See Figure 13-14.)

4. Exhale as you point your foot and slowly lower your leg to the floor, pressing your lower back and your right foot into the floor. Lower your leg to a point 1–2 inches above the floor and hold. Pause for a few breaths, squeezing your buttocks. (See Figure 13-15.)

5. Repeat steps 2–4 two more times. On the second lift, point and flex your foot. On the third lift, do ankle circles.

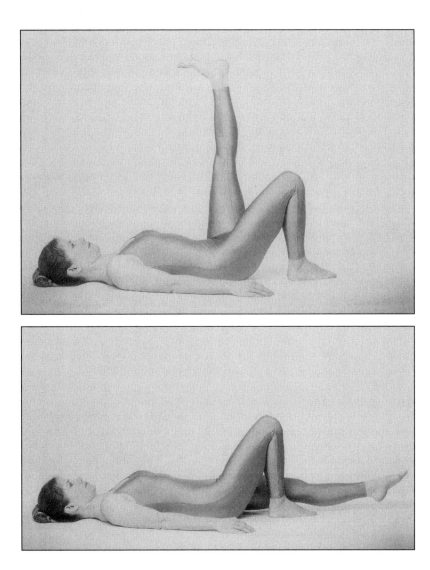

**Figure 13-14**
*As you lift your leg up to center, support your spine by pressing your lower back and right foot into the floor. Flex your foot and press it into the ceiling.*

**Figure 13-15**
*Lower your leg to a point 1–2 inches above the floor and hold. If your leg gets tired, send your breath to your muscles to energize them.*

6. Bring the left leg down to a resting position, sliding the right leg down to meet the left. Shake the legs out and rest for a few breaths.

7. Balance the body by repeating the sequence with the right leg. Close your eyes so you feel what's happening.

*continued*

**Figure 13-16**

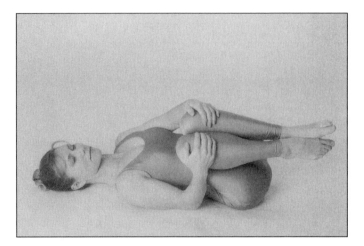

*Feel the pelvis being
engaged as you rotate
your knees around
in circles.*

## Counter Posture

Press your knees into your chest. Then with your hands
placed on your knees, rotate your knees around in circles. Feel the pelvis being engaged. (See Figure 13-16.) To
end, open your knees, allowing them to drop to the sides
by placing your soles together. Hold and rest.

# The Triangle Series (*Trikonasanas*)

The Triangle Series gives the body a complete side stretch as you form a triangle with your legs, arms, and torso. The series consists of the following three postures: Basic Triangle, Extended Triangle Pose, and Extended Side Angle Pose. They are explained and demonstrated on pages 148–154.

As you advance into the Extended Triangle, your hips, waist, abdominals, back, arms, and legs are strengthened and toned. You will find that doing this posture on a regular basis will help your body become stronger, you feel more balanced. Your ability to perform any posture is improved.

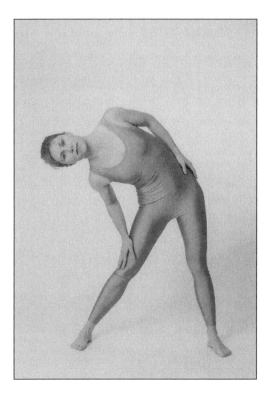

**Figure 13-17**

*Inhale and slide your right arm down the right side of the body, squeezing your buttocks to protect your spine.*

## Basic Triangle (*Trikonasana I*)

The full extension of the Basic Triangle gives your body an excellent full body side stretch in this first posture in the series.

1. Coming from a standing position, adjust your feet to be wider than shoulder width apart.

2. Inhale and slide your right arm down the right side of the body as far as is comfortable. (See Figure 13-17.) Squeeze your buttocks and hold for 10 breaths. Your knees are in a slight unlocked position.

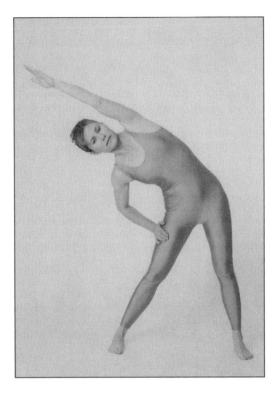

**Figure 13-18**

*Lift your left arm up and over, keeping it straight. Feel a deeper stretch along the left side of your body, especially in the hip and waist area.*

3. Come back up to center and rest for a few breaths.

4. Slide your right arm down your thigh again. Squeeze your buttocks and lift your left arm up and over your ear, keeping the arm as straight as you can. (See Figure 13-18.) Hold for 5 breaths.

5. Repeat on the left side.

### Focus

*To come out of this safely, lower your arm to your hips and keep your buttocks squeezed before standing up.*

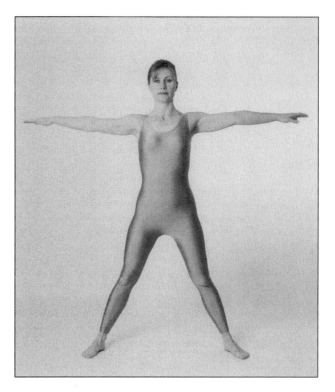

**Figure 13-19**

*Stand as tall as you can as you extend both arms out to the sides.*

## Extended Triangle Pose (*Utthita Trikonasana*)

You feel additional muscles and body parts being engaged in the Extended Triangle, especially the hamstrings, chest, arms, and shoulders.

1.  Come into a standing position. Adjust your feet to be wider than shoulder width apart. Extend both arms out to the sides. (See Figure 13-19.)

2.  Turn your right foot out to a 90-degree angle. Exhale and slide your right hand down to grab hold of your right foot or ankle. Lift your left arm up, palm facing forward. Turn your head and look up at your palm.

**Focus**

*Allow your left hip to come forward slightly to allow your upper body to bend down without bending your knee.*

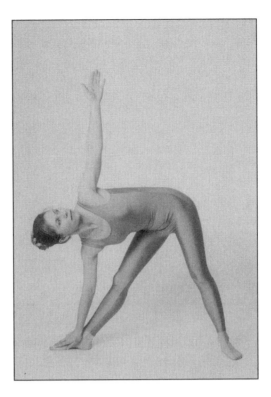

**Figure 13-20**

*Keep your extended arm straight and strong, lifting your fingertips into the ceiling. Your palm is flat, facing forward.*

(See Figure 13-20.) Keep your hips and pelvis facing forward. Squeeze your buttocks to protect your lower back. Hold for 10 breaths.

3. Lower your left arm down and lift the body back up to a standing position. Rest for a few breaths.

4. Repeat on your left side.

**Focus**

*If you can't reach your foot or ankle, grab your calf or wherever it is comfortable.*

**Figure 13-21**

*Work toward bending the leg so that your thigh becomes parallel to the floor. Ensure your knee is directly over your big toe for proper alignment.*

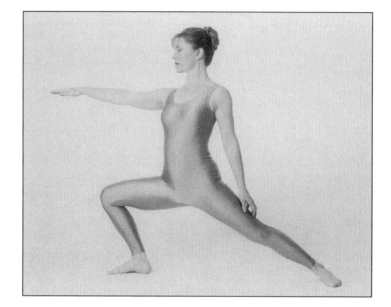

## Extended Side Angle Pose (*Utthita Parsva Konasana*)

A variation to the Extended Triangle, the Extended Side Angle Pose creates a deeper stretch along the side of the body, strengthening your calves, thighs, ankles, and knees, while stretching your waist and opening your hips. You will notice your balance being tested in this one as well. For deep toning in the thighs and buttocks, practice the advanced variation. This is the last posture in the Triangle Series.

**Extra Help**
*Grab hold of your calf or ankle if you cannot place the palm of your hand on the floor.*

1. Come into a standing position. Adjust your feet so they are wider than shoulder width. Turn your right foot out to a 90-degree angle. Turn your upper body to face your right foot as you bend your right knee, placing the knee directly over your big toe for proper alignment. Work toward bending the leg so that your thigh becomes parallel to the floor. Extend your right arm out, fingers pointed, palm down. (See Figure 13-21.)

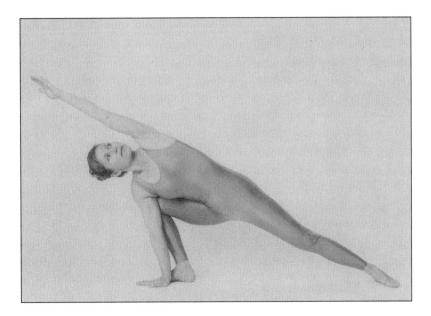

**Figure 13-22**

*Feel a complete lateral stretch in the full extension. Calm your breath as you breathe into the stretch, keeping your extended arm strong and straight.*

2. Lower your right hand, placing your palm on the floor next to your right foot. Lift and stretch your left arm up and over your head, palm down. Lower your arm toward your ear to form a diagonal line with your extended leg. Turn your head and look up at the ceiling. Hold for 10 breaths. (See Figure 13-22.)

3. To come out, lower your left arm down to your hips, straighten your right leg, and bring yourself back up to a standing position, with your arms at your side. Rest for a few breaths.

4. Repeat this sequence on your left side.

*continued*

### Focus

*Keep your extended arm as straight as you can. As soon as you feel the need to bend it, know you have stretched it far enough. Work toward getting it down to your ear while keeping it straight.*

**Figure 13-23**

*To start to get into the advanced stretch, bend down and place your right arm on the inside of your right leg, reaching back between your legs.*

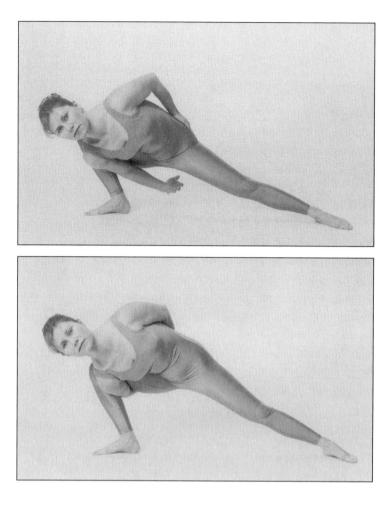

**Figure 13-24**

*Wrap your right arm around and up near your buttocks, reaching up to clasp your left hand behind you.*

## Advanced

This deep stretch is amazing for your buttocks and thighs, also giving your upper back, arms, and shoulders a nice stretch.

1. Coming from step 1, place your left hand on your lower back/buttocks. Bend down and place your right elbow on the inside of your right thigh. Begin to reach under your legs. Keep your head in alignment with your spine by looking ahead. (See Figure 13-23.)

2. Now wrap your right arm under your right leg and reach up your back to clasp your left hand. (See Figure 13-24.)

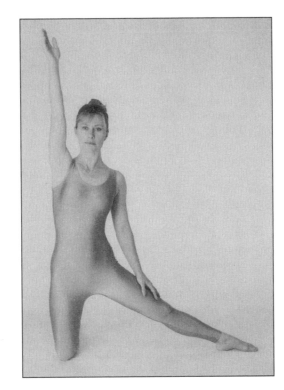

**Figure 13-25**
*Focus on your
extended arm,
keeping it as straight
as you can while
relaxing your neck.*

## Kneeling Side Stretch (*Parighasana*)

Feel your entire body being stretched as you arch from side to side. You especially feel energized in your upper body, arms, and shoulders as they too are being stretched, toned, and strengthened.

1. Come into a kneeling position, "standing" on your knees. Extend your left leg out to the side, foot pointed. Place your left hand on your left thigh. Lift your right arm up, keeping it as straight as you can while relaxing your neck. (See Figure 13-25.)

*continued*

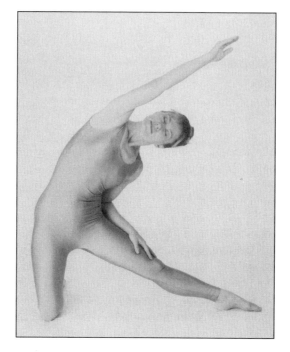

**Figure 13-26**
*Arch over to your left, creating a deep stretch along the right side of your body and up into your shoulders and arms.*

2. Arch over to your left, keeping your right arm straight. Lift your fingertips into the ceiling to help increase the stretch. Rest your left palm on your thigh. Stretch for 10 breaths. Close your eyes if you want to. Feel the stretch. (See Figure 13-26.) Come back to center.

3. As you come out of the stretch, keep your right arm extended and arch over to the right, placing your right palm on the floor. Lift your left arm up, keeping it strong and straight. (See Figure 13-27.)

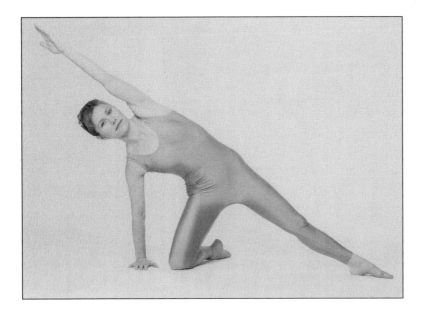

**Figure 13-27**
*Place your right palm
on the floor for a reverse
stretch. Feel a complete
lateral stretch.*

4. To come out of this safely, lower your arm down first,
   squeeze your buttocks, and center, standing on your
   knees again. Pause for a few breaths.

5. Repeat with extending your right leg out, lifting your
   left arm up.

**Figure 13-28**

*Focus on your arm as you sit up tall and straight. Relax your neck as you try and place your arm close to the side of your head while keeping it as straight as possible.*

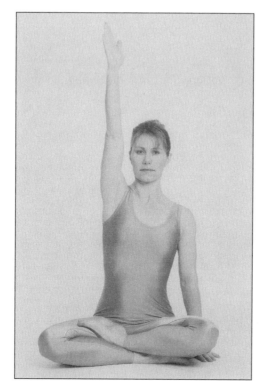

## Seated Side Stretch

The Seated Side Stretch is a variation to the Kneeling Side Stretch. As in the kneeling version, the side of your body is stretched, in this one, from your buttocks up into your arm.

1. Come into a comfortable sitting position instead of standing on your knees. Lift your right arm up, keeping it as straight as you can while relaxing your neck. Place your left palm on the floor at your side. (See Figure 13-28.)

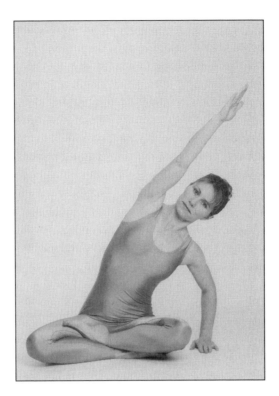

**Figure 13-29**
*Arch over to your left. Feel a stretch from your buttocks, into your hips, waist, up into your underarm, and the entire length of the arm. Press your left palm into the floor for support.*

2. Arch over to your left. The position of the extended arm does not change. Lift your fingertips into the ceiling, keeping your right sitting bone pressed into the floor. (See Figure 13-29.) Stretch for 10 breaths. Come back to center and lower your arm.

3. Repeat with the left arm.

**Figure 13-30**

*Feel your hips open as you allow your knees to drop to the side. As you breathe, your body relaxes into the posture.*

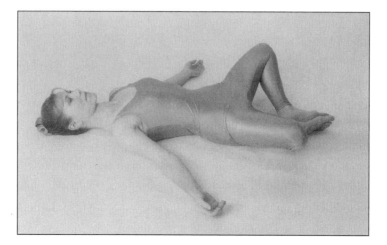

## Goddess Pose (*Supta Baddha Konasana*)

The Goddess Pose is an "open life" posture, opening you up as your knees drop to the side. You feel vulnerable and exposed. Know that when you create, these two qualities are important. As you breathe in, you begin to feel more comfortable and more at ease with yourself as you are exposed. You relax into the posture. Take this lesson and use it in your life whenever you are feeling vulnerable.

Do this posture last in your series of the second chakra postures. A lot of issues may come to the surface, wanting to be released. Acknowledge their presence and let them go.

*Note:* This is also a wonderful posture to do during pregnancy.

1. Come into a lying position with your knees bent. Place the soles of your feet together as you press your lower back into the floor. Allow your knees to drop to the sides. Completely relax your legs, allowing them to drop further. Stretch your arms out to the side of your body. (See Figure 13-30.)

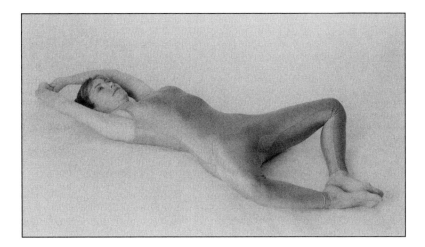

**Figure 13-31**
*For a further release,
bring your arms up
over your head.*

2. Hold this position for a count of 10 breaths. As you breathe in, your body relaxes into the posture.

3. To end, bring your arms up over your head and clasp your hands. Stretch your body to release any further energy needing to be released. Hold for 5 breaths. (See Figure 13-31.)

4. Bring your knees back together and stretch the legs out.

## Comfort Aid
*If you can't clasp your hands together, try holding on to a towel to achieve the same stretch, or simply leave your hands where they can comfortably reach and work toward stretching them further.*

Chapter 14

# Chakra Three Postures

Come back and center, bringing your focus inward. Perform this brief meditation to help activate the energy of your third chakra. Become aware of the body parts involved in this chakra, along with the emotional meaning attached to it. The chakra continues to open and balance as you engage in the following postures.

*You now move up into your third energy center. Breathe in and thank the orange ray as you leave it and move into your Divine Power, your Solar Plexus center. Your third energy center is located at your abdominal area. You are in your power and at peace here. You see a bright sunshine yellow. Visualize a band of sunshine yellow in the front and behind your third energy center to help activate it.*

*As you enter this energy center, center yourself and ask that you release any emotional element that no longer serves your purpose and affirm:*

*"I feel my feelings."*

*This is where you house the powerful energy of your emotions and feelings, and where you act on those feelings. Your third energy center has to do with the use of your personal power and it is here you experience the action of breaking away from societal beliefs, where you let go of attachments and feel comfortable with yourself for doing so. This energy is strong and positive, connecting you to the world around you.*

*The postures for your third energy center are designed to strengthen your Solar Plexus, your Power and Emotional center, to help you become more of an observer in situations instead of getting "pulled" in to other's energy.*

*Breathe in the sunshine yellow. Feel its energy as you explore the body parts that affect your power and your emotions.*

# Abdominal Strengthening Series

Your emotional body is directly linked to your physical body. When you are weak on a physical level you are weak in your corresponding emotional body, and vice versa.

This is especially true in your Solar Plexus, your emotional and power center, where you store your energy, your power, and your emotions.

Weakened abdominal muscles translate to a weakened emotional body. Women must take care, especially after their childbearing years when the abdominal muscles are weakened, to strengthen these muscles so that you remain strong emotionally and in your power.

Strong abdominal muscles are important for proper body alignment and are required in order to perform most yoga postures safely and efficiently. Although not part of a traditional yoga program, I add them to my daily routine to help protect my body.

The following series of four postures gently strengthen your Solar Plexus: Half Sit-Up, Goddess Pose Sit-Up, Extended Leg Sit-Up, and Open "V" Sit-Up. These are explained and demonstrated on pages 166–172.

Throughout these postures, concentrate on using your abdominal muscles to lift the upper body while relaxing your neck and shoulders.

## Half Sit-Up

1. Come into a lying position with your knees bent. Place your hands on your upper thighs. (See Figure 14-1.)

2. Inhaling, slide your hands up your thighs until you can look over your knees. (See Figure 14-2.) You are lifting your upper body by using your abdominal muscles. Keep your head in alignment with your spine. Press your lower back into the floor. Relax your neck and shoulders. Hold for 5 breaths.

3. Lie back down. Rest for a few breaths. Your feet remain on the floor with your hands at your sides.

4. Repeat 2 more times.

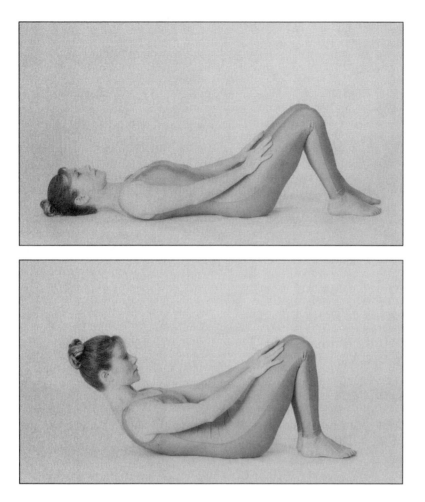

**Figure 14-1**
*Bend your knees and place your hands on your thighs.*

**Figure 14-2**
*Keep your neck in alignment with your spine as you lift your upper body by using your abdominals. Remember to breathe.*

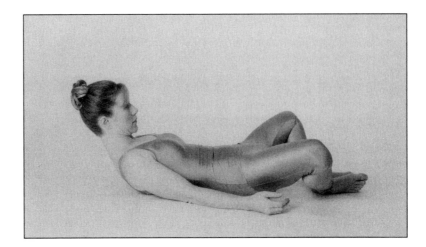

## Goddess Pose Sit-Up

Move into the Goddess Pose following the Half Sit-Up. Focus on your abdominal muscles as you lift your upper body.

1. Lie on the floor with your knees bent. Place the soles of your feet together, allowing your knees to drop to the sides. Inhale and lift your upper body, using your abdominal muscles. (See Figure 14-3.) Relax your neck and shoulders, consciously not engaging these body parts. Hold for 5 breaths.

2. Exhale and lower your upper body down. Bring your knees into your chest and press them into your chest for a few breaths to release your lower back.

3. Repeat 2 more times.

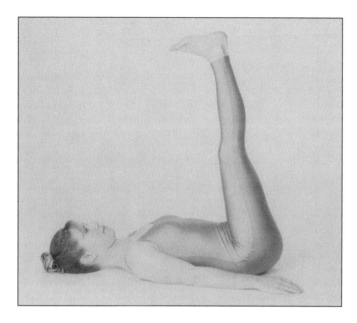

**Figure 14-4**
*Extend both legs
up while pressing
your lower back into
the floor. Begin
to focus on your
abdominal muscles.*

## Extended Leg Sit-Up

Continue the flow of the Abdominal Strengthening Series. Again, focus on your abdominal muscles as you lift your upper body, breathing throughout these exercises. Feel these muscles being engaged as you relax your neck and shoulders, keeping your head in alignment with your spine.

1. Come into a lying position with your knees bent. Extend both legs up, keeping them as straight as possible while pressing your lower back into the floor. (See Figure 14-4.)

2. Inhale and lift your upper body, using your abdominal muscles. Allow your arms to float along the side of your thighs. Your head is in alignment with your spine. Relax your neck and shoulders as you pull your upper body up. Hold for 5 breaths. (See Figure 14-5, page 170.)

*continued*

**Figure 14-5**

*Keep your neck in alignment with your spine as you lift using your abdominal muscles. Press your lower back into the floor.*

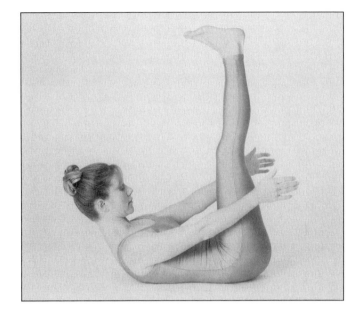

3. Exhale and lower your upper body down. Bring your knees into your chest and press them into your chest for a few breaths to release your lower back.

4. Repeat 2 more times.

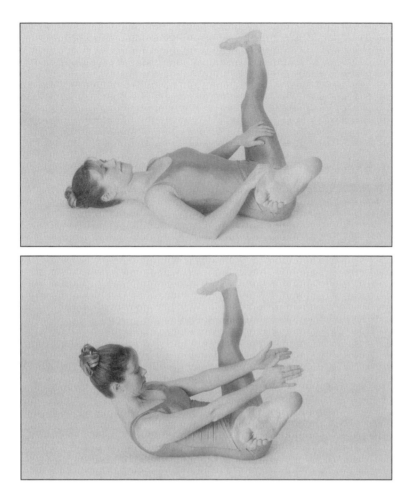

**Figure 14-6**
*Open your legs into a "V," pressing your lower back into the floor. Begin to focus on your abdominal muscles.*

**Figure 14-7**
*Extend your arms inside the "V" as you lift your upper body. Press your lower back into the floor. Remember to breathe.*

## Open "V" Sit-Up

Continue the flow from the Extended Leg Sit-up. Focus on the muscles being used as you relax your neck and shoulders, keeping your head in alignment with your spine. This ends the Abdominal Strengthening Series.

1. Come into a lying position with your knees bent. Extend both legs up and open them into a "V," pressing your lower back into the floor. Rest your hands on the inside of your thighs. Keep your feet flexed. (See Figure 14-6.)

*continued*

**Figure 14-8**

*Imagine pulling a rope
to strengthen your
outer abdominal
muscles.*

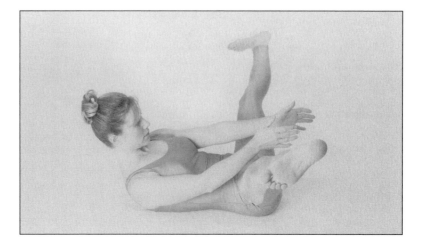

2. Extend your arms inside the "V." Inhale and lift your upper body, using your abdominal muscles. (See Figure 14-7, page 171.) Press your lower back into the floor. Relax your neck and shoulders, keeping your head in alignment with your spine. Hold for 5 breaths.

3. Now imagine your hands holding a rope as you pull the rope toward you. Continue pulling for 5 breaths. (See Figure 14-8.)

4. Exhale and lower your upper body down. Bring your legs together. Bend your knees into your chest, pressing them into your chest for a few breaths to release your lower back.

5. Repeat 2 more times.

## Counter Posture

Press your knees into your chest. Rotate your knees from side to side as you gently massage your lower back. Both shoulders remain on the floor.

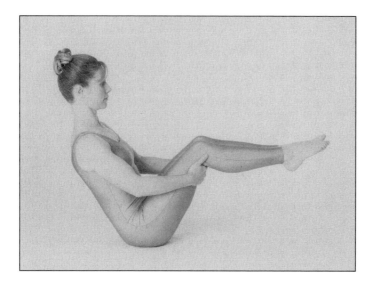

**Figure 14-9**
*Lift your feet off the floor and lower your upper body to form one-half of the "V." Lift your spine to help straighten your back.*

## Upward "V" Posture or Boat Posture (*Paripurna Navasana*)

In this traditional yoga posture, the body forms a "V" shape or boat, strengthening your abdominal muscles as it holds the body in position. This posture is one of your more difficult postures to get into, mostly because it requires strong abdominal muscles to maintain the balance required. The Boat works your upper and lower abdominal muscles, as well as your thighs and upper back. Progress through this one slowly and carefully, being careful not to strain your lower back.

1. Come into a sitting position with your knees bent. Place your hands under your knees. Lift your feet off the floor so that your calves are parallel to the floor. Lower your upper body backward slightly, forming half of the "V." (See Figure 14-9.)

*continued*

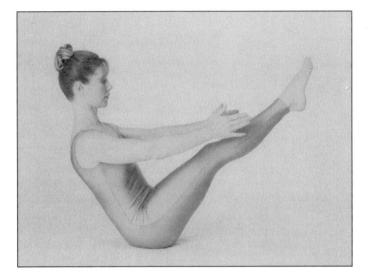

**Figure 14-10**

*Extend your legs to form the "V." Lift your spine and your legs, tensing your thighs to help keep your legs in position.*

2. Extend your legs up and out to form the second half of the "V." Extend your arms straight ahead, palms facing each other. Look at your feet. (See Figure 14-10.) Do not collapse your lower back and do not tense your abdomen. Hold this position for 5 breaths.

3. Exhale and lower your legs to the floor to protect your lower back. Hug your knees.

4. Repeat 2 more times.

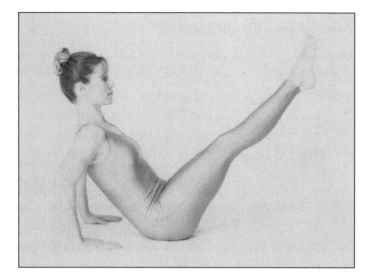

**Figure 14-11**
*For added support, place your hands on the floor behind you.*

## Variation

For added support, in step 2, place your hands on the floor behind you as you extend your legs. (See Figure 14-11.) Do this until your abdomen is strong enough to support your upper body on its own.

## Bow Pose (*Dhanurasana*)

Do the Bow Pose after the Abdominal Strengthening Series or the Boat posture to help stretch out your abdominal muscles. This posture strengthens your Solar Plexus, your center that stores all your energy. Your Solar Plexus needs to be cleaned out of the negative energy holding you back. It is also an excellent choice for stretching your thighs, opening the chest, and awakening the spine.

1. Come into a tummy position. Reach back and grab hold of your ankles as you bring both feet toward your buttocks. Your knees are shoulder width apart. Press your abdomen into the floor. Keep your face down, but not resting on the floor. Relax your neck and shoulders. (See Figure 14-12.)

2. Inhale and lift your body by squeezing your shoulder blades together. Feel your chest opening. Press your ankles into your hands to allow your legs to be lifted higher. Feel the stretch in your thighs. Look straight ahead and breathe deeply into your chest for 5 breaths. (See Figure 14-13.)

3. Lower your arms and legs. Place your hands shoulder width apart, and turn your head to the side to relax your neck.

4. Repeat 2 more times.

### Counter Posture

Go into the Child Pose. (See Figures 10-1 and 10-2, page 89.)

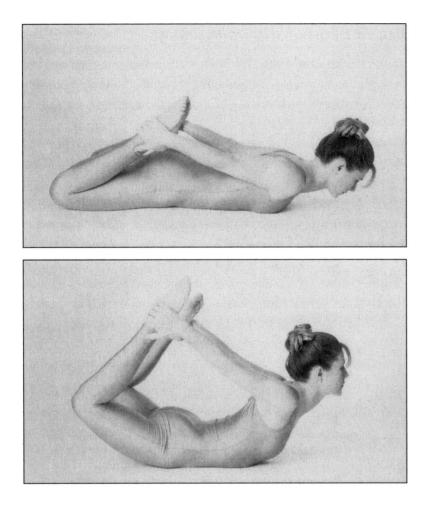

**Figure 14-12**
*Keep your face down, but not resting on the floor as you grab your ankles.*

**Figure 14-13**
*Lift your upper body by squeezing your shoulder blades together. Lift your lower body by pressing your ankles into your hands.*

## Warrior Pose (*Virabhadrasana*)

**Focus**

*Do not bend your leg down parallel to the floor if this is too difficult. Only go down as far as is comfortable. Advance into getting the thigh parallel as your thigh strengthens.*

Named after a powerful mythological warrior, this posture not only strengthens your physical body but is placed in the third chakra postures for its empowering qualities as you work and strengthen your Power and Emotional center.

As you stand and center, focus on doing your actions in this world, staying in your heart and staying in your third chakra, allowing your actions to reflect love and understanding, empowering yourself. The Warrior Pose teaches you to move from a place of power into a place of expression, moving from the heart and a place of empathy while staying centered in your power.

As you do this posture, keep your eyes open, because you want to "know" what you are doing. Feel the empowerment. As you advance through the positioning of the Warrior, you stretch and strengthen your entire body, with particular emphasis on your thighs.

1.  Come into a standing position. Adjust your feet so they are wider than shoulder width apart. Extend your arms to the side and look straight ahead. (See Figure 14-14.)

2.  Turn your left foot out to a 90-degree angle. Bend your left leg to form a 90-degree angle, your knee in alignment with your toes. Your thigh is parallel to the floor. Arms remain extended to both sides with your right hip staying back. Use your right foot as a support to the extended leg. (See Figure 14-15.) Hold for 5 breaths. Work toward holding the Warrior for 3 minutes on each side.

3.  Move directly into the four variations that follow at your own pace, relaxing your bent leg by straightening it as needed.

4.  After the variations, stand and rest for a few breaths. Repeat with the other leg.

*continued*

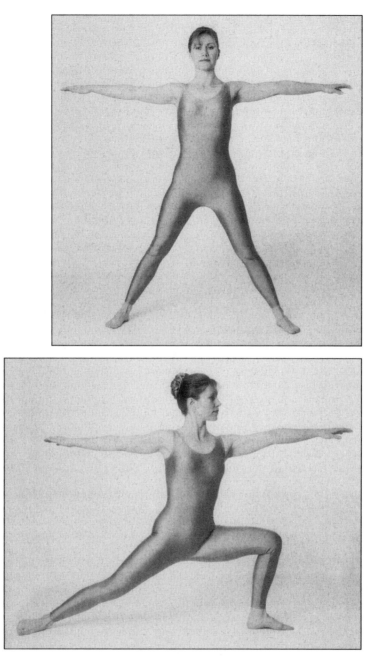

**Figure 14-14**
*Extend your arms to the side as you stand as tall as you can. Relax your neck as you stretch your arms out.*

**Figure 14-15**
*Keep your thigh parallel to the floor, with your shin perpendicular. Keep the arms straight and strong. Extend your upper body up.*

**Figure 14-16**

*Turn your upper body to face your bent knee. Place your hands in the prayer position.*

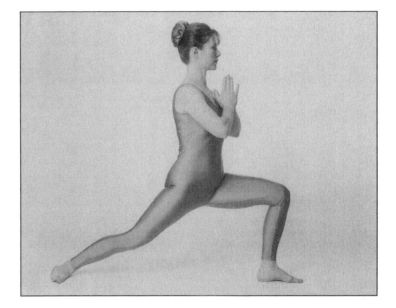

**Focus**

*Straighten your bent leg for a few breaths if it tires, then lower it down again as you continue through the posture.*

## Variation I

From step 2, turn your upper body to face your bent knee. Place your hands in the prayer position over your heart. Square your hips forward, supporting your extended leg with your left foot. Try to keep your right heel down. Hold for 5 breaths. (See Figure 14-16.)

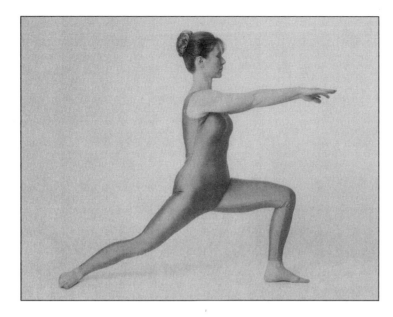

**Figure 14-17**
*Extend your arms out
as if lunging, relaxing
your neck. Remember
to breathe.*

## Variation II

From step 2, extend your arms straight ahead as if
lunging. Keep your arms as straight as you can while
relaxing your neck and shoulders and keeping your head
in alignment with your spine. Square your hips forward,
supporting your extended leg with your left foot. Try to
keep your right heel down. Hold for 5 breaths.
(See Figure 14-17.)

*continued*

> **Extra Help**
> *Allow your arms
> to rest down at
> your side if
> needed as you
> progress through
> the Warrior.*

**Figure 14-18**

*Extend your arms up, palms facing each other. Keep them as straight as you can while relaxing your neck. Look straight ahead or up at your palms, whichever is easier on your neck.*

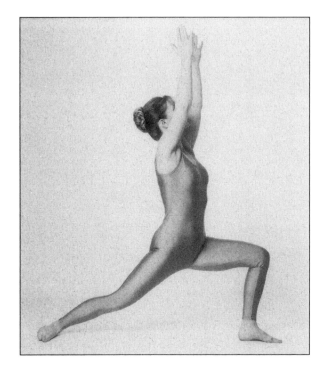

## Variation III

From step 2, extend your arms straight up, palms facing each other. Keep your arms as straight as you can while relaxing your neck and keeping your head in alignment with your spine. Look straight ahead or up at your palms. Square your hips forward, supporting your extended leg with your left foot. Try to keep your right heel down. Hold for 5 breaths. (See Figure 14-18.)

### Focus

*Alternate between variations as it suits your needs. Hold each variation for 5 breaths. Work toward holding the Warrior for 3 minutes on each side, while alternating through the variations.*

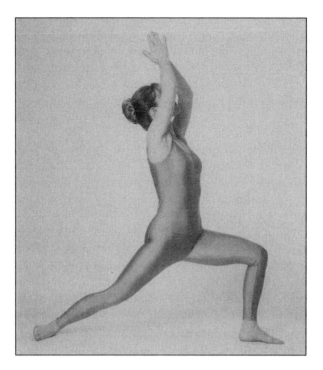

**Figure 14-19**
*Place your palms together and look up at them. Feel the difference in the upper arms and neck. Be careful not to tense your neck muscles.*

## Variation IV

From Variation III, place the palms of your hands together and look up at your palms. Remember to breathe as you relax your neck and allow your head to drop back. Hold for 5 breaths. (See Figure 14-19.) This is more difficult than it looks.

Chapter 15

# Chakra Four Postures

Bringing your focus inward, perform the following brief meditation to help activate the energy of your fourth chakra. Become aware of the body parts involved in this chakra, as well as the emotional meaning attached to it. This chakra continues to open and balance as you engage in the following postures.

*You now move up to your fourth chakra, your Heart chakra. As you leave the yellow ray, you also leave your three lower chakras and move up into your Heart chakra. There are three chakras below and three chakras above the Heart chakra. You must pass through your Heart chakra to get to either location. This is why the heart is placed where it is. You are in the middle, the center of your humanness. This is the place you learn forgiveness, compassion, love, and discernment. This is where you learn your lessons.*

185

*Your fourth chakra is located from the base of your rib cage all the way up to the base of your throat, including your arms and hands. Relax your body, allowing your breath to go deeply into all parts of the body. Feel your shoulders dropping down in front of your ears. Your hands are relaxed and open to receiving knowledge. You receive gifts from your hands. You exchange hugs and greetings with your hands.*

*As you move into your Heart chakra, you see a beautiful emerald green. Visualize the emerald green in the front and behind your fourth energy center and affirm:*

*"My heart is open."*

*Feel the energy of the emerald green.*

*While in this place, scan your body to see if you are predominately a giving person or a receiving person. To balance the Heart chakra, open yourself up to receiving if you are predominately a giving person. Imagine yourself receiving gifts. If you are predominately a receiving person, open up to be a giving person. Step out of your safety, that place of familiarity, and invite the other energy in, to balance.*

*Visualize your Heart chakra opening so that you can feel love and compassion. Strengthen your Heart chakra now that it is open.*

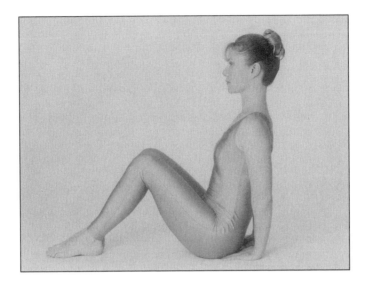

**Figure 15-1**

*Place your fingertips under your buttocks to help support your spine and buttocks when in the full extension of the posture.*

## Fish Posture (*Matsyasana*)

The Fish Posture teaches you to open your Heart chakra so that you are in a receptive place—you are able to receive. This posture opens your upper chest and shoulders as you arch your back. It also loosens the hip joints and stretches the upper thighs as you allow the knees to drop open, opening all the chakras as you do so.

1. Come into a sitting position with your knees bent. Place your fingertips under your buttocks. (See Figure 15-1.)

2. Exhale and lower your upper body onto your elbows, lifting your chest up as you gently lower your head back, placing the crown of your head on the floor. (See Figure 15-2, page 188.) Hold for 5 breaths.

*continued*

### Focus

*When your head is lowered back, always protect it when coming out of the position by lifting your head as a separate movement.*
*In this posture, lift your head up first **before** coming up into a sitting position.*

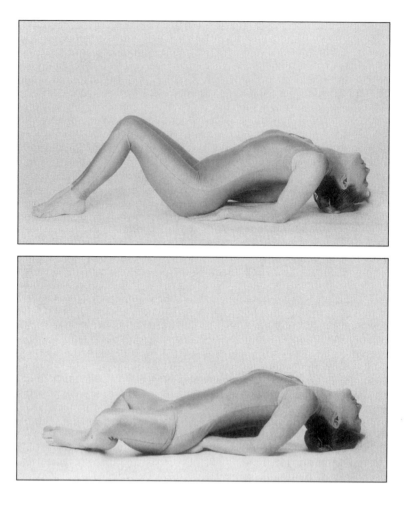

**Figure 15-2**

*Lift your chest up as you gently lower your head back, placing the crown of your head on the floor. Allow your elbows, not your head, to take the weight.*

**Figure 15-3**

*Open your legs, allowing the knees to drop to the floor, completely relaxing your body.*

3. Open your legs, allowing the knees to drop to the floor, completely relaxing your body. (See Figure 15-3.) You are opening all your chakras as your entire spine is exposed. Squeeze your buttocks to protect the lower back as you hold for 5 breaths.

4. To release, exhale and lift your head first to protect your neck. Bring your knees together and slide the legs back down. Come back into a sitting position.

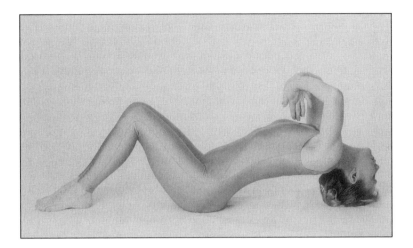

**Figure 15-4**
*Keep the palms together and turn the hands down, lowering your hands until your fingers touch your chest.*

## Advanced Fish I

This variation allows for flexibility in your wrists as the energy moves down into your Heart center.

1.  Coming from step 2, extend your hands to the side and lift them up over your chest, keeping them as straight as possible, until your palms touch together in the prayer position. Keep the palms together and turn the hands down, lowering your hands until they touch your chest. Hold for 10 breaths. (See Figure 15-4.)

2.  Release your arms and bring them down to the side of your hips. Exhale and lift your head and come back into a sitting position.

*continued*

**Figure 15-5**

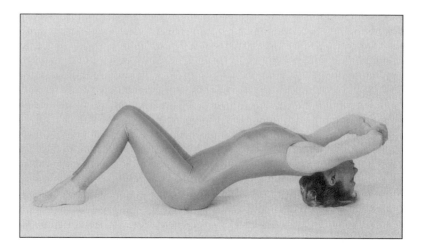

## Advanced Fish II

This variation requires flexibility in your shoulders and may take some time to master. The added stretch expands the chest further, increasing the capacity of the rib cage and lungs.

1. Coming from step 2, clasp your arms together, bending at your elbows. Stretch your clasped arms over your head, trying to place them on the floor. (See Figure 15-5.) Hold for 10 breaths. Look up toward your forehead.

2. Release your hands and place them back under your buttocks. Exhale and lift your head first and then come back up into a sitting position.

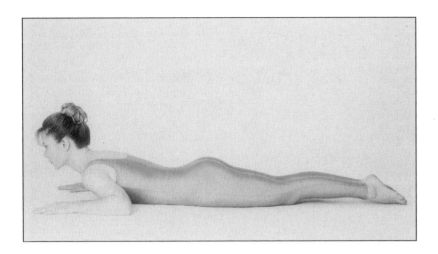

**Figure 15-6**

*To begin this posture, lift your upper body without putting any pressure on your hands. Squeeze your buttocks to support your lower back. You should feel no strain.*

## Cobra (*Bhujangasana*)

Feel the body expanding as it stretches like a rubber band into the Cobra. Whenever you do the Cobra, feel how deeply you drop inward and gain access to that place of stillness because your heart is open. Open your chest as you feel the energy moving from your open heart all the way up to your Third Eye. The powerful Cobra strengthens your back as it opens your chest.

1. Come into a tummy position. Place your hands on the floor, wherever it is comfortable, to begin the posture.

2. Squeeze your buttocks, and without pressing your hands into the floor, gently lift your upper body off the floor while focusing on your lower back. (See Figure 15-6.) You are simply allowing your body a chance to respond to the full extension of the posture.

3. Lower the body down with your head resting to one side. Rest for a few breaths.

*continued*

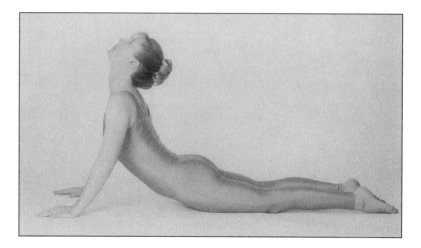

**Figure 15-7**

*Squeeze your buttocks and gently lift your upper body off the floor by pressing your hands into the floor. Keep your elbows slightly bent. Breathe into the chest as you feel it opening.*

4. To come into the full extension of the Cobra, adjust your hands so they are even with and close to the shoulders. Breathe and press your hands into the floor, lifting your upper body as you squeeze your buttocks together. Keep your elbows slightly bent to protect your lower back, concentrating on using your back muscles to lift your upper body from the floor. Keep your head held, yet lowering it back just enough to be able to look up at the ceiling. Drop your shoulders down, opening your chest. Hold for 10 breaths. (See Figure 15-7.)

5. Slowly lower the upper body down, with the head the last to come down. Come down as gracefully as you came up. Rest the head to one side for a few breaths while relaxing your arms.

6. Repeat 1 more time.

## Counter Posture

Come into the Child Pose. (See Figures 10-1 and 10-2, page 89.)

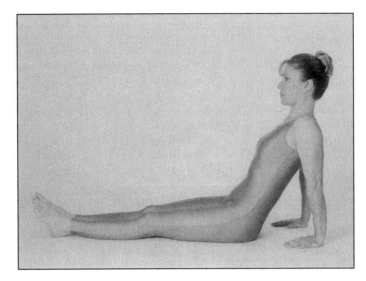

**Figure 15-8**

*Place the palms of your hands behind your buttocks, about six inches away, with your fingertips facing your buttocks.*

## Plank Posture

Feel your shoulders and chest open as you stretch your body into the Plank Posture. Your body literally takes the form of a "plank" as you hold this position, strengthening your hands, wrists, arms, shoulders, stomach, and buttocks. Squeeze your shoulder blades together to help support the body and help take the weight off of your hands and wrists.

1. Come into a sitting position with your legs extended in front of you. Keep your back/spine as straight as possible. Place the palms of your hands behind your buttocks, flat on the floor, about six inches away. Your fingers are pointing toward your buttocks. (See Figure 15-8.)

*continued*

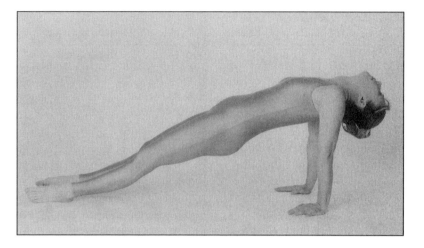

**Figure 15-9**

*Squeeze your buttocks as you lift your hips square into the ceiling. Squeeze your shoulder blades together to support your body. Keep your legs and arms straight.*

2. Inhale and lift your body as you allow your head to drop back. Point your toes. Squeeze your buttocks as you lift your hips square into the ceiling. Support your body with your arms. Keep your legs and your arms straight as you press your chest and hips into the ceiling. (See Figure 15-9.)

3. Hold for 5 breaths. Release by lowering your buttocks to the floor, and gently lift your head to come back into a sitting position.

4. Repeat two more times.

## Counter Posture

From the sitting position, slide your knees into your chest and hug them.

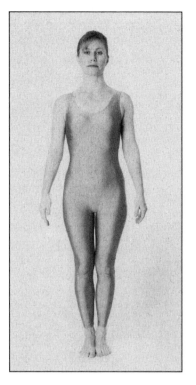

**Figure 15-10**

*As you stand as tall as you can, imagine your head being pulled up by a string, encouraging your spine to straighten further.*

## Mountain Posture (*Tadasana*)

The Mountain Posture is the basic standing pose in yoga. It allows you to stand straight and tall while realigning the spine for proper posture.

1. Come into a standing position, consciously standing as straight and tall as you can. Place your feet together with your arms at your sides. Begin breathing through your nostrils. (See Figure 15-10.)

*continued*

2. Inhale and begin lifting your arms, palms up, stretching them out from your side. Relax your neck and shoulders. Continue to slowly lift your arms until the palms of your hand touch.

3. Press the palms of your hands together while relaxing your neck and shoulders. You won't be able to press very hard. Look straight ahead, calming your breath. Imagine a string attached to your fingertips. Imagine someone pulling up on this string to encourage your spine to straighten further. Breathe in and out as you straighten your arms as far as is comfortable. (See Figure 15-11.)

4. Look up at your palms to release your neck as you relax your neck, shoulders, and upper back. Hold for 10 breaths. (See Figure 15-12.)

5. Exhale and lower your hands down to your side. Pause and center for a few breaths.

6. Repeat 2 more times.

## Counter Posture

Shake your shoulders out or come down into the Elephant Posture (pages 128–130) if you feel the need to release your lower back, upper back, or neck muscles.

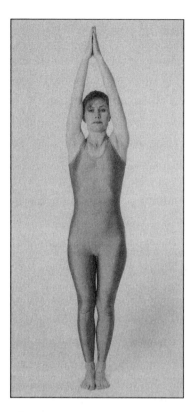

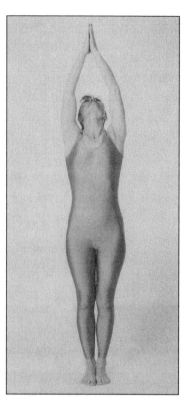

**Figure 15-11**

*Press the palms of your hands together while consciously relaxing your neck. Imagine your fingertips are being pulled by a string, lengthening your spine further.*

**Figure 15-12**

*Look up at your palms to release your neck.*

## Standing Chest Opener (*Tadasana II*)

The Standing Chest Opener is an ideal posture to include in your daily routine as it releases stress and tension in your upper back and shoulders—a place that stress seems to rest in all us. Feel yourself being grounded in the full extension of this posture as you stand for a moment with an open heart. This is where your power comes from—from being in your heart.

This movement opens the chest while releasing the neck and throat area. Adjusting your feet to a comfortable standing position and keeping your knees in an unlocked position will protect your lower back.

1. Coming from the Mountain Posture (Figure 15-10, page 195), adjust your feet to slightly less than shoulder width apart. Extend your arms out in front of you. Keep your knees in a slightly unlocked position. (See Figure 15-13.)

2. Swing your arms around the sides of your body and all the way around to the back. Roll and squeeze your shoulder blades as you clasp your hands together. Squeeze your buttocks and allow your knees to bend slightly to protect your lower back. (See Figure 15-14.)

*continued*

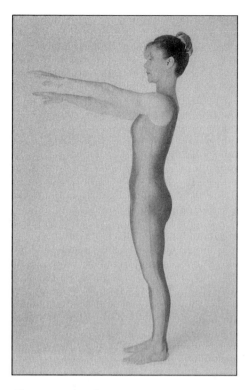 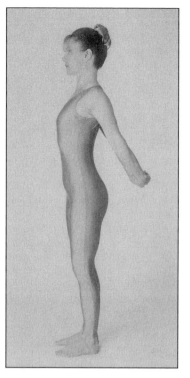

**Figure 15-13**

*Extend your arms out in front of you, relaxing your shoulders.*

**Figure 15-14**

*Roll and squeeze your shoulder blades together as you clasp your hands behind you. Unlock your knees to take any strain off of your lower back.*

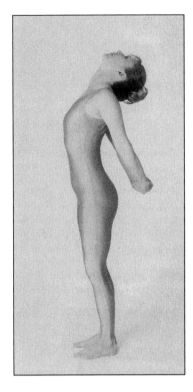

**Figure 15-15**
*Feel a deeper stretch as you lower your head back.*

3. Inhale, and as you exhale, lower your head back. Open your chest as you continue to squeeze your shoulder blades. Lower your head as far as is comfortable, completely letting your neck muscles release. Hold for 10 breaths. (See Figure 15-15.)

4. Release your hands and bring them down to a resting position. Exhale and gently lift your head up and rest for a few breaths.

5. Repeat 2 more times.

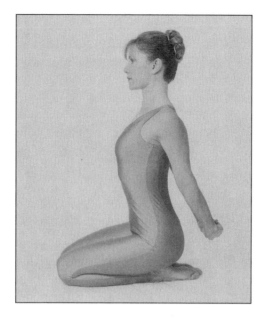

## Sitting Chest Opener

Developed as a variation to the Standing Chest Opener, this flow of postures further works to open your Heart chakra. As you sit, squeeze your shoulder blades back to engage your heart. Release when you feel your heart open. Your heart is where you get your confidence. You feel strong when you come from an open heart. This series of movements stretches the neck and lower back, and opens the chest to encourage deep breathing.

1. Come into a kneeling position, your feet and knees are together as you sit on your heels. Begin breathing through your nostrils. Squeeze your shoulder blades back, clasping your hands behind you. Keep your arms straight as you pull down on your arms, opening your chest. Inhale and arch your spine. Hold for 5 breaths. (See Figure 15-16.)

*continued*

**Figure 15-17**

*Extend your arms up behind you as you squeeze your shoulder blades together. Feel a stretch in the upper back and upper arms.*

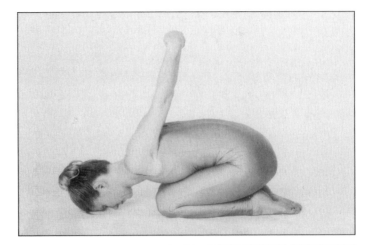

**Figure 15-18**

*Roll your buttocks up, placing the crown of your head on the floor. Feel your spine being stretched with a deeper stretch in your arms as you lock them back.*

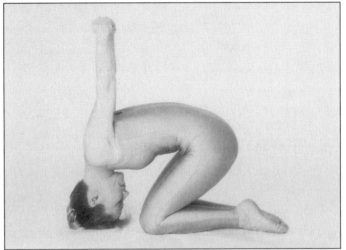

2. Exhale and bend your upper body forward, coming down into the Child Pose. Extend your arms up behind you as you squeeze your shoulder blades together. Your hands remain clasped behind your back with your forehead resting on the floor in front of your knees. Hold for 5 breaths. (See Figure 15-17.)

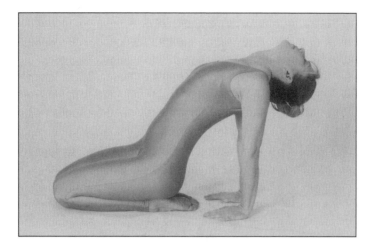

**Figure 15-19**

*As a reverse stretch, arch back, lowering your head back. Lift your chest into the ceiling as you release your neck.*

3. Roll forward, placing the crown of your head onto the floor. Inhale and lift your buttocks, raising your clasped hands up to the ceiling. Hold for 5 breaths. (See Figure 15-18.)

4. Come back into the kneeling position. Place your hands behind you, palms down, with your fingers facing your buttocks. Inhale and lower your head back, lifting and opening your chest. Breathe deeply into your chest for 5 breaths as you completely let go of your neck. (See Figure 15-19.)

5. Straighten your body back up into a kneeling position before lifting your head. Exhale and lift your head.

### Focus

*When your head is lowered back, always protect it when coming out of the position by lifting your head as a separate movement. Come back into a kneeling position first **before** lifting your head.*

# Wrist Circles with Extended Arms (*Tadasana III*)

Your arms are an extension of your Heart chakra—you give and receive with your arms and hands. In this posture, your arms are extended to receive healing from your heart. Feel the energy moving through your arms and into your hands. The energy you feel comes from your Heart chakra. When completed, feel the difference in your arms.

This posture strengthens your upper back, shoulders and arms. It stretches your arms and wrists and energizes your hands and fingers. Adjusting your feet to shoulder width will give you the proper balance to extend your arms to the side.

1. Coming from the Mountain Posture (Figure 15-10, page 195), adjust your feet to shoulder width apart. Your hands are at your sides, palms up. Inhale and lift your arms to shoulder height. Relax your neck and consciously open your chest as you squeeze your shoulder blades together. Squeeze and hold for 3 breaths. (See Figure 15-19.)

2. Release your arms and bring them down to your side. Relax for a few breaths. Feel your arms relax, feeling the relaxation leaving through your fingertips.

3. Inhale and lift your arms up again, palms up. Begin wrist circles, 10 in each direction. Relax your neck and shoulders as you continue breathing in and out. (See Figure 15-20.)

4. Release your arms and bring them down to your side.

## Counter Posture

Do the Standing Chest Opener, dropping your head back to release tension in your neck. (See pages 198–200.)

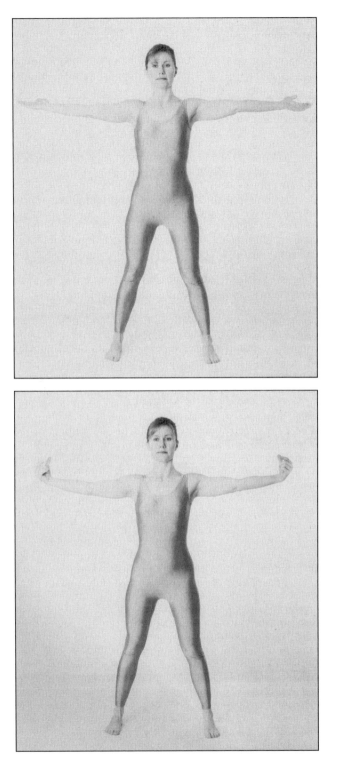

**Figure 15-19**
*Consciously open your chest as you squeeze your shoulder blades together.*

**Figure 15-20**
*Relax your neck and shoulders as you perform wrist circles in both directions.*

## Camel Posture (*Ustrasana*)

**Focus**

*When your head is lowered back, always protect it when coming out of the position by lifting your head as a separate movement. Straighten your spine, coming out of the arch, **before** lifting your head.*

This is one of my favorite postures because of its releasing benefits in the upper back and neck area. The Camel is also included in the fifth chakra postures as it is equally beneficial in opening your Throat chakra as it is in opening your Heart chakra.

1. Come into a kneeling position with your arms at your sides.

2. Place your hands behind you, supporting your upper body on your fingertips. Inhale and squeeze your shoulder blades as you gently lower your head back, completely allowing the neck to release. (See Figure 15-21.) Breathe through your nostrils as you arch your back, lifting and opening your chest. Hold for 10 breaths.

3. Exhale and lift your head up. Bring your arms back to your sides and rest for a few breaths.

4. Repeat 2 more times.

### Variation

If your knees are bothered by a kneeling position, come into a sitting position in step 1, with your legs extended in front of you. Continue on to step 2. (See Figure 15-22.)

*continued*

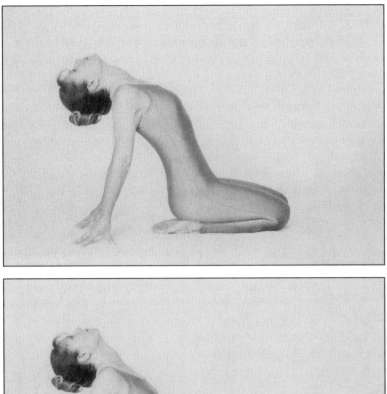

**Figure 15-21**
*Inhale and squeeze your shoulder blades as you gently lower your head back, allowing the neck to release. Lift your chest into the ceiling.*

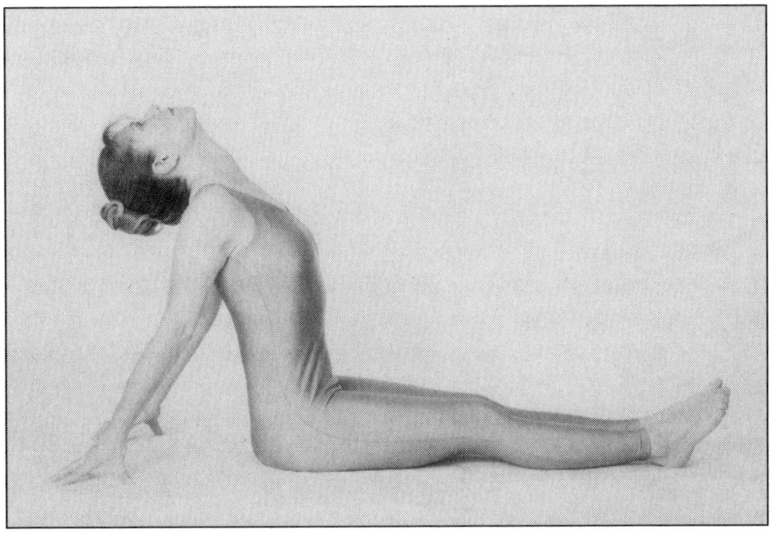

**Figure 15-22**
*As a variation, extend your legs out in front of you instead of kneeling.*

## Advanced

### Extra Help

*As your body becomes more limber, inch your hands down your feet and onto the floor to increase the stretch.*

1. Come into a standing position on your knees with your arms at your sides. Look straight ahead. Adjust your knees so that they are a little wider than shoulder width apart. (See Figure 15-23.)

2. Bring your arms around behind you and grab hold of your heels. Press your palms into your heels as you lower your head back. Squeeze your shoulder blades together and lift your chest up, gently lowering your head and completely allowing your neck to release. Press your hips and pelvis forward as you arch your back to achieve the full extension of this posture. (See Figure 15-24.) Feel the stretch in your thighs. Squeeze your buttocks to protect your lower back. Hold for 10 breaths. As your body becomes more limber, inch your hands down your feet and onto the floor to increase the stretch.

### Focus

*When your head is lowered back, always protect it when coming out of the position by lifting your head as a separate movement. Straighten your body back up into the kneeling position **before** lifting your head.*

3. Straighten your body back up into the kneeling position before lifting your head. Exhale and lift your head. Bring your arms back to your sides and rest for a few breaths.

4. Repeat two more times.

## Counter Posture

Come down into the Child Pose. (See Figures 10-1 and 10-2, page 89).

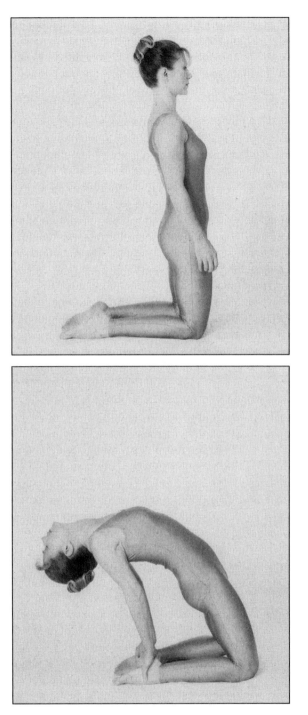

**Figure 15-23**
*Come into a standing position on your knees with your arms at your sides.*

**Figure 15-24**
*Press your hips and pelvis forward as you arch your back to achieve the full extension of this posture.*

## Cow-Head Pose (*Gomukhasana*)

### Comfort Aid

*If you have difficulty sitting up straight, sit on two or three folded towels or blankets.*

*If you have difficulty clasping your fingers, grab hold of a belt or towel.*

The Cow-Head Pose opens the entire chest area as it limbers your shoulders, upper back, and upper arms. If you cannot grasp your fingertips together, try holding on to a towel until your shoulder muscles loosen up enough for your fingers to touch.

1. Come into a comfortable sitting position. Bring your right hand behind you, palm out, reaching to the top of your back as high as you can. Stretch your left arm up toward the ceiling. (See Figure 15-24.)

2. Bend your left arm at the elbow and bring it down to touch your upper back. Clasp your fingertips together. Breathe into your chest as it opens. Hold for 10 breaths. (See Figure 15-25.)

3. Release your arms and rest for a few breaths.

4. Repeat, alternating your arms.

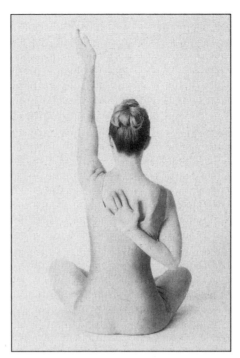

**Figure 15-24**
*Reach to the top of
your back with your
right hand and stretch
your left arm up.*

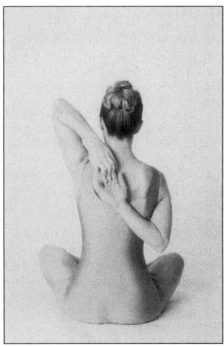

**Figure 15-25**
*Clasp your fingertips
together and breathe
into your chest
as it opens.*

Chapter 16

# Chakra Five Postures

Bringing your focus inward, perform this brief meditation to help activate the energy of your fifth chakra. You become aware of the body parts involved in this chakra, as well as the emotional meaning attached to it. This chakra continues to open and balance as you engage in the following postures.

*As you give thanks and leave your Heart chakra, you move up along your spine to your fifth energy center, your Throat chakra. You see the color of the sky—sky blue. Consciously place this mass of blue energy into your Throat chakra. It shimmers with the Truth, the courage to speak your truth. The blue energy vibrates out, covering your neck and chin, your jaws, cheeks and nose, your ears and eyes, in the front and behind, and you affirm: "My throat is open," or "I speak my truth." Feel the energy.*

*And now, open the body parts of your Throat chakra. While you are sitting, lower your jaws to relax them. Relax your entire body. The intention of this is to help you see what you need to remove and be aware of in order to have your throat more open and to speak your truth from your heart. Ask the question, "What is it that needs to be removed from my Throat chakra so I may speak freely?" Allow a word or sentence to come. Acknowledge it and let it go.*

*Breathe deeply. Feel the powerful energy of the sky blue. Innately do one of the fifth chakra postures your body needs. This will help you loosen the energy blocks. Continue to do the postures you feel your body needs. If you feel the need, do them all. Use your breath to deepen and release. You are fully protected. Allow your body to open.*

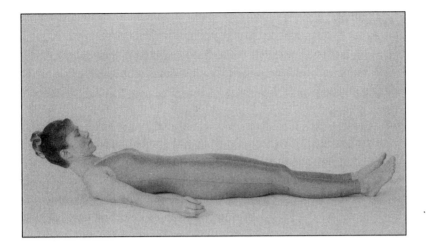

## Neck Lifts

The Neck Lifts gently strengthen weak neck muscles. This posture is useful when recovering from a neck injury.

1. Come into a lying position. Relax your entire body.

2. Inhale and gently lift your head as high as is comfortable. (See Figure 16-1.) Breathe through your nose as you hold this position for for 3 breaths. As your neck strengthens, work up to holding for 10 breaths.

3. Lower your head and rest for a few breaths.

4. Repeat 2 more times.

## Camel Posture (*Ustrasana*)

### Note

*Refer to chapter 15, "Chakra Four Postures," for photos.*

### Focus

*When your head is lowered back, always protect it when coming out of the position by lifting your head as a separate movement. Straighten your body back up into the kneeling position **before** lifting your head.*

This is one of my favorite postures because of its releasing benefits in the upper back and neck area. The Camel is included here in the fifth chakra postures as well as in the fourth chakra because it is equally beneficial in opening your Throat chakra as it is in opening your Heart chakra.

1. Come into a kneeling position with your arms at your sides. Look straight ahead.

2. Place your hands behind you, supporting your upper body on your fingertips. Inhale and squeeze your shoulder blades as you gently lower your head back, completely allowing the neck to release. (See Figure 15-21, page 207.) Breathe through your nostrils as you arch your back, lifting and opening your chest. Hold for 10 breaths.

3. Exhale and lift your head up. Bring your arms back to your side and rest for a few breaths.

4. Repeat 2 more times.

### Variation

If your knees are bothered by a kneeling position, come into a sitting position in step 1, with your legs extended in front of you. Continue on to step 2. (See Figure 15-22, page 207.)

### Advanced

1. Come into a standing position on your knees with your arms at your side. Look straight ahead. Adjust your knees so that they are a little wider than shoulder width apart. (See Figure 15-23, page 209.)

2. Bring your arms around behind you and grab hold of your heels. Press your palms into your heels as you lower your head back. Squeeze your shoulder blades together and lift your chest up, gently lowering your head and completely allowing your neck to release. (See Figure 15-24, page 209.) Press your hips and pelvis forward as you arch your back to achieve the full extension of this posture. Feel the stretch in your thighs. Squeeze your buttocks to protect your lower back. Hold for 10 breaths. As your body becomes more limber, inch your hands down your feet and onto the floor to increase the stretch.

3. Straighten your body back up into the kneeling position before lifting your head. Exhale and lift your head. Bring your arms back to your sides and rest for a few breaths.

4. Repeat 2 more times.

## Counter Posture

Come down into the Child Pose. (See Figures 10-1 and 10-2, page 89).

**Extra Help**
*As your body becomes more limber, inch your hands down your feet and onto the floor to increase the stretch.*

# Rabbit Posture

The Rabbit Posture compensates for the backward arch of the Camel Posture, while it limbers up your spine before entering the Shoulder Stand. Feel the stretch in the upper back and shoulders as you roll forward.

1. Come into a kneeling position and lower your upper body until your forehead touches the floor (this is the Child Pose). Grab hold of your heels or the outside of your feet. Keep your forehead on the floor and your buttocks on your feet. Relax your shoulders, neck, and face as you breathe into your chest. (See Figure 16-2.)

2. Now place the crown of your head onto the floor. Touch your forehead as close as possible to your knees. If you can't touch your forehead to your knees, walk your knees up to your forehead. Continue to hold on to your heels. (See Figure 16-3.)

3. Lift your buttocks as you round your back, holding onto your heels. Feel the stretch in the upper back and shoulders. Hold this position for 20 breaths, being careful not to rest your weight on your head. Support yourself with your arms by pulling on your heels. (See Figure 16-4.)

4. Let go of your heels and come down into the Child Pose.

5. Repeat 2 more times.

## Counter Posture

Stay in the Child Pose until your spine is rested.

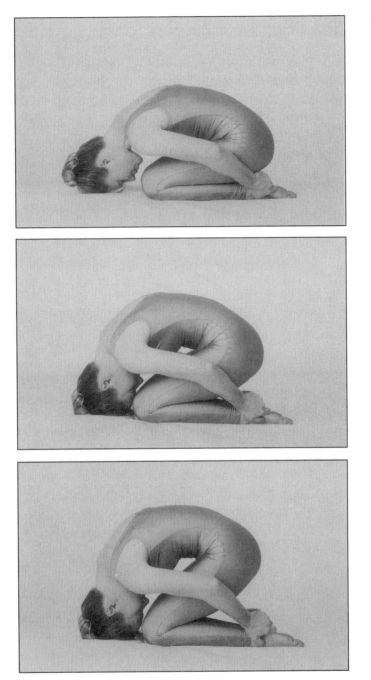

**Figure 16-2**
*Grab hold of your heels or the outside of your feet. Begin to feel a stretch in your upper back and arms.*

**Figure 16-3**
*Place the top of your head on the floor. Walk your knees up to your forehead if they are not touching. Continue to breathe into your chest.*

**Figure 16-4**
*Lift your buttocks as you round your back, feeling a deep stretch in the upper back and shoulders. Continue to breathe.*

# Shoulder Stand Series (*Sarvangasana*)

This series of postures is called the "queen" or "mother" of all the postures because it works the "whole body," the literal translation in Sanskrit. You don't want to miss out on the rejuvenating effects of this flow of postures. The Shoulder Stand and Plough will completely energize your body, with the added benefit of relieving fatigue and premature aging.

The Shoulder Stand Series is another one of my favorites and it is wise to include them in your daily routine of yoga. These postures stretch out your limbs and your entire spine from the base of your neck all the way down to your tailbone, stretching all the muscles along the spine. Progress from one posture to the next as your spine becomes more flexible.

The series consists of the following three postures: Half Shoulder Stand, Shoulder Stand to Plough Pose, and Advanced Plough. These are explained and demonstrated on pages 221–227.

Allow for the transition of going into the Shoulder Stand and the Table before going into the Plough Pose. This prevents muscles along your spine from being pulled and/or strained, protecting your spine from injury. Smoothly move into the Plough by allowing your feet to drop to the floor, and only when your body is ready for this added stretch.

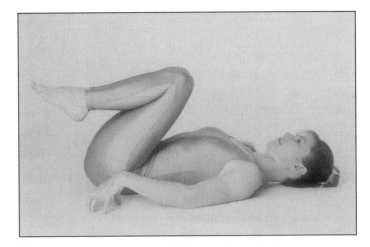

## Half Shoulder Stand (*Ardha Sarvangasana*)

1. Come into a lying position with your knees bent. Place your fingertips on the floor, allowing them to act as a springboard. Press your knees into your chest. (See Figure 16-5.)

2. Inhale and lift your buttocks off the floor and extend your legs. Lower your legs to a 45-degree angle into the Half Shoulder Stand. Support your lower back with your hands, or if it is easier, continue to press your hands into the floor. Keep your legs as straight as possible. (See Figure 16-6, page 222.) You are not trying to touch your toes to the floor behind you at this point. Relax your upper back and hold for 10–20 breaths. Go directly into the full Shoulder Stand from here when you are able.

> ### Comfort Aid
> *If you experience tightness in your neck or upper back area, place 2 or 3 blankets under your shoulders and arms, with your head on the floor to help support your neck.*

*continued*

**Figure 16-6**

*Lower your legs to a 45-degree angle into the Half Shoulder Stand. Support your lower back with your hands.*

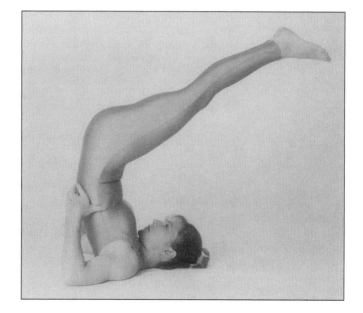

### Focus

*Pay attention to your lower back when coming out of the posture when using the support of blankets because your lower back is now lifted off the floor, making it more difficult to gently roll out of the posture.*

3. Exhale and gently lower your knees back into your chest, rolling your body down vertebra by vertebra, until you come back down into a lying position

4. Relax for a few breaths, then repeat 2 more times.

## Variation

If you are having trouble getting into the Half Shoulder Stand, position yourself against a wall. In step 1, place your buttocks as close to the wall as possible. Push off against the wall into position.

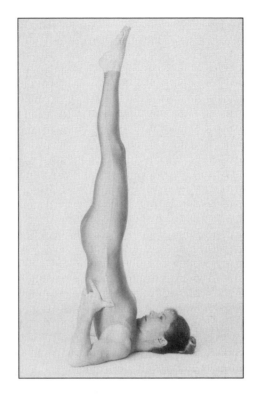

**Figure 16-7**
*You are trying to keep your legs in alignment with your spine, your body perpendicular.*

## Shoulder Stand to Plough Pose (*Salamba Sarvangasana Halasana*)

Flow into the full Shoulder Stand from the Half Shoulder Stand when you feel strong enough. You will need to engage your abdominal muscles in order to safely support your body while in the Shoulder Stand.

1. Coming from step 1 for the Half Shoulder Stand (see Figure 16-5, page 221), lift your legs straight up toward the ceiling. Place your hands on your lower/middle back to support your body, squeezing your buttocks. Consciously relax your neck as it begins to stretch in this posture. You are trying to keep your legs in alignment to your spine. You will need to use your abdominal muscles to help you do this, while continuing to squeeze your buttocks to support your lower back. Hold this position for 10–20 breaths. (See Figure 16-7.)

*continued*

**Figure 16-8**

*Bring your legs down, keeping your legs as straight as possible and parallel to the floor. This is referred to as the Table.*

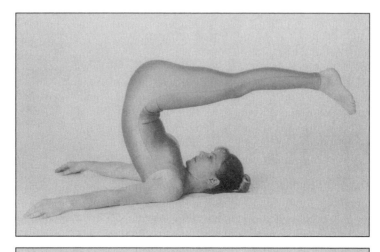

**Figure 16-9**

*Exhale and slowly lower your feet toward the floor into the Plough Pose. Feel the stretch along the spine, upper back, and into the neck.*

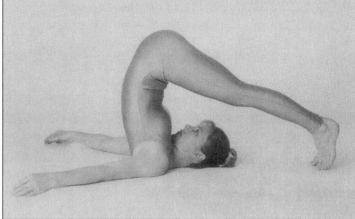

**Comfort Aid**

*If you have difficulty placing your toes on the floor, rest your toes on a couple of towels or blankets.*

2. Exhale and bring your legs down into the Table position, keeping your legs as straight as possible and parallel to the floor. (See Figure 16-8.) Hold for 30 breaths. Allow your arms to rest comfortably on the floor.

3. Exhale and slowly lower your feet toward the floor into the Plough Pose, only if this feels comfortable. (See Figure 16-9.) Hold for 10–20 breaths. Move into the Advanced Plough (page 226) from here when you are ready.

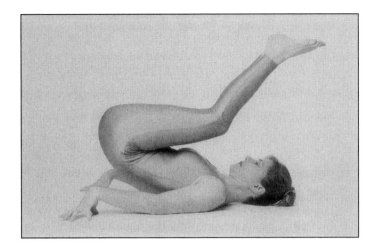

4. To come out of the Plough or Shoulder Stand, bend your knees down into your chest, rolling your body down vertebra by vertebra. (See Figure 16-10.) Roll down until you come into the Relaxation Posture (see Figure 4-2, page 23).

5. Relax for a few breaths, then repeat 2 more times.

## Focus

*If you feel **any** strain in your neck or spine you are not ready for the Plough. Go back to the Table and gently work toward bringing your toes down. Be careful not to push yourself from this point on as it is very easy to pull a muscle along the spine if your muscles aren't flexible enough yet.*

## Advanced Plough (*Karnapidasana*)

When you feel you have comfortably mastered the Plough, you are ready to move into the Advanced Plough. Feel a deeper stretch along the entire length of your spine, the back of your neck, upper back, and shoulder blades. Come out of this posture slowly and gently. You will lose many of the benefits achieved in this posture as well as injure your spine if you bring your body out of this posture too quickly.

1. Come into the Advanced Plough directly from the Plough Pose (step 3, page 224). Bend your knees into the floor, completely relaxing your neck as you do so. Hold this position for 10–20 breaths. (See Figure 16-11.)

2. To come out of the Advanced Plough, gently roll your body down until you are able to bend your knees into your chest, rolling your body down vertebra by vertebra. (See Figure 16-10, page 225.) Roll down until you come into the Relaxation Posture (see Figure 4-2, page 23).

3. Relax for a few breaths, then repeat 2 more times.

### Counter Posture

Continue to relax in the Relaxation Posture. Innately go into any other stretches or counter postures your body needs. Some suggestions are the Knee to Chest Posture (pages 60–61) or the Knee Down Twist (pages 62–63).

### Extra Help

*As your spine loosens and becomes more flexible, gently push on your lower back, gently pushing your knees further into the floor. Do this only as you progress through this posture, and only as your comfort level permits.*

### Comfort Aid

*To help you advance in to the Advanced Plough, place your knees on a of couple towels or blankets.*

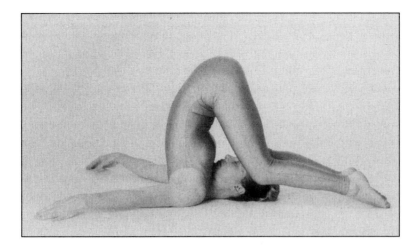

**Figure 16-11**

*Bend your knees into the floor, completely relaxing your neck as you do so. Remember to breathe.*

**Figure 16-12**
*Inhale and bring your chin down to your chest.*

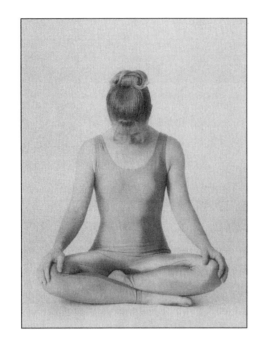

## Neck Rolls

Allow your Throat center to open as you relax your jaws through this posture. These rolls release tension in your neck and upper back while stretching the muscles all around the neck. When you have completed the Neck Rolls from side to side, pause for a moment before dropping your head back. Feel the back of the neck releasing as you open the Throat center at the back.

1. Come into a comfortable sitting position, sitting up as straight as possible. Your head is in alignment with your spine, and yours hands are on your knees or thighs. Inhale, and bring your chin down to your chest. (See Figure 16-12.)

2. Roll your head to the right, trying to place your right ear on your right shoulder. Relax the jaws. Hold for 5 breaths. (See Figure 16-13.)

3. Roll your head forward, bringing your chin back down to your chest. Pause for a few breaths.

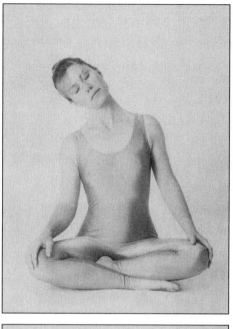

**Figure 16-13**

*Roll your head to the right, trying to place your right ear to your right shoulder. Gently pull down on the left shoulder to help increase the stretch.*

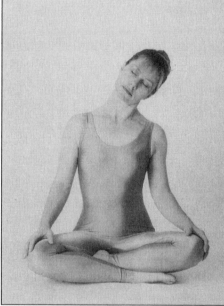

**Figure 16-14**

*Place your left ear to your left shoulder, gently pulling down on the right shoulder.*

4. Continue to roll your head around, trying to place your left ear on your left shoulder. Hold for 5 breaths. (See Figure 16-14.)

*continued*

**Figure 16-15**
*Inhale and gently lower your head back. Calm your mind and emotions as you completely release your neck. Allow your mouth to open to relax your jaw.*

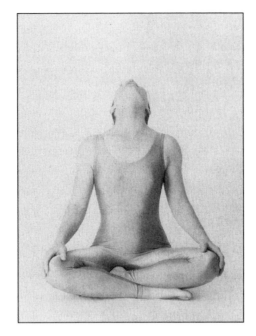

### Focus

*Always lower your head back as a separate movement from the side to side neck rolls, consciously being aware as you gently lower the head back to prevent injury.*

5. Bring your head up to center and rest for a few breaths, breathing deeply to relax your entire body.

6. Repeat steps 2–5, rolling your head to the left side, repeating the cycle

7. Inhale and gently lower your head back, if you can. Open your Throat chakra as you lift your chest up. Open your mouth to relax your jaw. Continue to breathe in and out, holding this position for 5 breaths. (See Figure 16-15.)

8. Lift your head up and center.

Chapter 17

# Chakra Six Postures

The sixth energy postures help strengthen your Third Eye, your forehead, as you learn to still your mind so that your focus can become clear and balanced. These postures will strengthen your physical body, but they are used here to strengthen your Third Eye. Still your mind and stay focused in these postures, without losing concentration or balance. When your mind is clear and balanced, your physical body becomes still and balanced as well.

Perform this brief meditation before going into the postures to help activate the energy of your sixth chakra. Become aware of the body parts involved as well as the emotional meaning attached to it. This chakra continues to open and balance as you engage in the postures.

*As you move up from your fifth energy center, thank and acknowledge the blue ray for allowing you to speak up freely. Look up and see a bright indigo blue color. You are entering your sixth energy center known as your Third Eye.*

*The Third Eye represents a higher vibration, a higher mind beyond structure as compared to the first center. As you come into your Third Eye, you use discernment. You consciously know this is a finer vibration. You have moved into your place of your "inner knowing," your center of intuition and inspiration. It is here that you are able to access your inner knowledge as you open your Third Eye to "see" and "know" intuitively. You affirm to yourself:*

*"I am intuitive. I am willing to 'see' and 'know' the truth."*

*From here you benefit from being "in the moment," because when you live in the moment, fear does not enter in. Fear comes from your logical mind and when you let it in, it takes you "out" of the moment. It is said that living in the moment takes the stress out of your life because you no longer need to fear what happened in your past or what may happen in your future. The finer vibration of the Third Eye will guide you. It uses its own laws, its own knowingness.*

*Honor your intuition as your sixth energy center grows in strength and intensity. It is here that you learn to trust that area of the unknown, but now with using discernment. It is about living in the moment, without fear, trusting yourself and opening yourself to seeing new possibilities and other perspectives. When you honor your "self" and others, you come from your higher "self," your knowing "self." You are moving toward wholeness, which is "self."*

*Trust yourself to open up and be still. Stand and center for a moment, breathing in the indigo blue light as you feel your inner eye opening to access your intuition, allowing you to look into your future. Feel the energy of the indigo blue.*

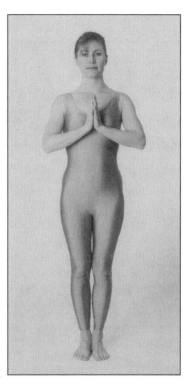

**Figure 17-1**
*Place your hands in the prayer position. Close your eyes and ask your mind to be still.*

## Tree Pose (*Vrksasana*)

The object of this pose is to help you find and hold your center. You learn to still your mind and calm your breath, focusing on your breath to help keep you in your center. Placing your hands in the prayer position will calm you and help you focus inward. As you stand in this Candle position, allow your inner light to shine brightly. This pose develops mental balance as well as physical balance. As you progress, you will find it easier to calm your mind and gain better control of your balance.

1. Come into a standing position. Place your hands in the prayer position over your heart. Feel your inner light shining brightly. Focus on your breath to help you find and hold your center. (See Figure 17-1.)

*continued*

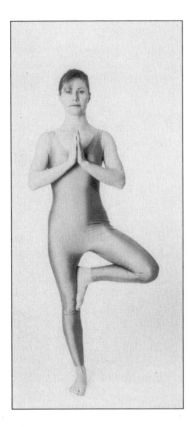

**Figure 17-2**

*Place your left foot on the inside of your right thigh as high as is comfortable.*

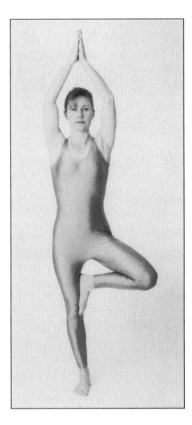

**Figure 17-3**

*Raise your arms up over your head until your palms touch.*

2. Fix your attention onto a spot directly ahead of you, as you slide your left foot and place it on the inside of your right thigh. Place your foot as high as is comfortable. (See Figure 17-2.)

3. When you feel you are properly balanced, raise your arms up over your head until your palms touch. Bend your elbows slightly, relaxing your neck and shoulders. Look straight ahead. (See Figure 17-3.) Continue to focus on your breath as you hold this posture for 10 breaths. If you feel you are well balanced, try closing your eyes while holding this posture. If you lose your balance, go back to step 2 to regain your focus and try again.

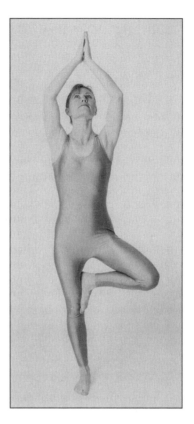

**Figure 17-4**
*Look up at the palms of your hands and continue to focus on your breath.*

4.  If you can, look up at the palms of your hands and continue to focus on your breath as you hold this posture for 10 breaths. (See Figure 17-4.)

5.  Lower your arms and your foot and come back into a standing position. Rest for a few breaths.

6.  Repeat this sequence on your opposite leg.

## Focus

*For added balance, extend your arms out to the side if you wish. If needed, place your foot anywhere along the inside of the opposite leg, even balance your foot against your ankle with your toe on the ground for a starting position if you like.*

## Standing Bow (*Natarajasana*)

Despite its difficulty, the Standing Bow is one of the more beautiful and graceful poses in yoga. It is a pose worth striving to perfect not only for its grace, but also for its aspects of balance, flexibility, coordination, and strength. The Standing Bow opens your hip joints while stretching and strengthening the muscles in your lower back, chest, abdomen, buttocks, and legs, especially the upper thighs. The Standing Bow symbolizes a constant flow of energy as it allows for a complete stretch, improving the spine's flexibility. As you fully extend your body in this posture, imagine your body arching like a strung bow.

1. Come into a standing position, and center with your eyes closed. Open your eyes and fix your gaze on a spot directly ahead of you. Balancing on your right leg, bend your left leg back and grab hold of your foot with your left hand, on the inside or the outside, whichever is most comfortable. (See Figure 17-5.)

2. Extend your right arm up. Hold for a few breaths while you gain your balance. (See Figure 17-6.)

*continued*

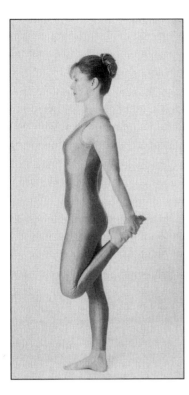

**Figure 17-5**

*Balancing on your right leg,*
*bend your left leg back and*
*grab hold of your foot with*
*your left hand.*

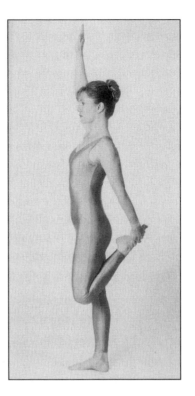

**Figure 17-6**

*Extend your right arm up*
*and hold while you gain*
*your balance.*

**Figure 17-7**

*Maintain alignment of your extended arm, neck, spine, and thigh throughout the posture. Stay calm as you try to lift your leg higher by pressing your foot into your hand.*

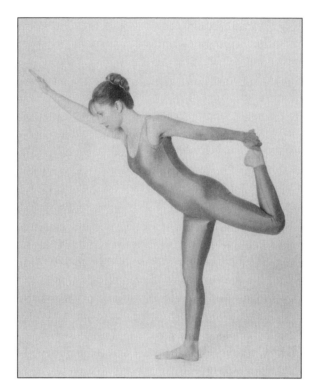

3. Lower your upper body until your thigh, spine, neck, head, and right arm are in a straight line. Your fingertips are in alignment with the top of your head, palm down. (See Figure 17-7.) Allow your eyes to drop to the floor. Press your left foot into your hand to help you lift the leg higher. Keep your gaze fixed to the floor and hold this position for 10 breaths. Breathe normally, relaxing your breath, as your stretch forward as far as you can for a complete body/spine stretch.

4. Slowly release and pause for a few minutes before repeating on the opposite side.

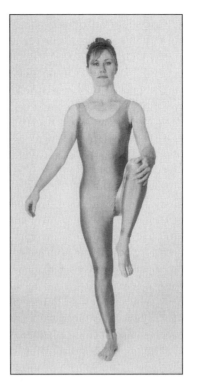

**Figure 17-8**

*Bring your left knee into your
chest and steady your balance.*

## Dancer's Pose Balancing Posture (*Utthita Hasta Padangusthasana*)

Named after a pose a dancer would perform, this posture strengthens the legs and hips while using the element of balance. You learn to clear your mind and focus your attention in order to develop balance and a sense of calm. This posture opens the hip area as you swing the bent leg out to the side, strengthening your hips while toning the legs. The advanced extension stretches the entire length of your leg and opens the hips further.

1. Come into a standing position with your feet shoulder width apart. Your spine is completely straight and erect. Find a focal point ahead of you. Bring your left knee up into your chest, holding it with your left hand until you have steadied your balance. (See Figure 17-8.)

*continued*

Chakra Six Postures • 239

2. Firmly plant your right foot into the floor. Spread your toes apart for additional support. Slowly swing your left leg out to the side. Balance yourself with your right arm. (See Figure 17-9.)

3. When you have mastered your balance, look over your left shoulder. Hold for five breaths. (See Figure 17-10.)

4. Repeat on the other side.

*continued*

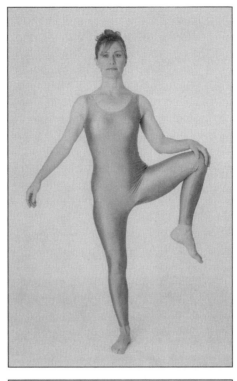

**Figure 17-9**
*Swing your left leg out to the side, balancing with your right arm.*

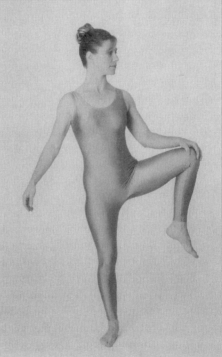

**Figure 17-10**
*When you have mastered your balance, look over your left shoulder.*

**Figure 17-11**

*Grab your big toe on your left foot with your left hand.*

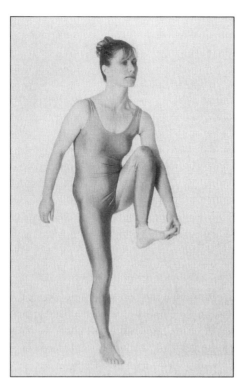

## Advanced

1. Coming from step 1, grab your big toe on your left foot with your left hand. (See Figure 17-11.)

2. Inhale and fully extend your leg out in front of you. (See Figure 17-12.)

3. Keeping your hips and shoulders facing forward, slowly swing your left leg out to the side. (See Figure 17-13.)

4. When you have mastered your balance, look to your left shoulder. Hold for five breaths.

5. Repeat on the other side.

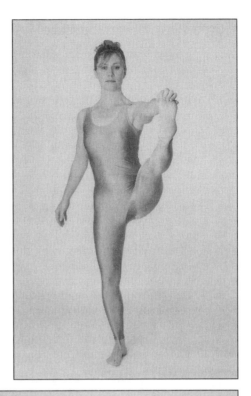

**Figure 17-12**
*Inhale and fully extend your leg out in front of you. Remember to breathe.*

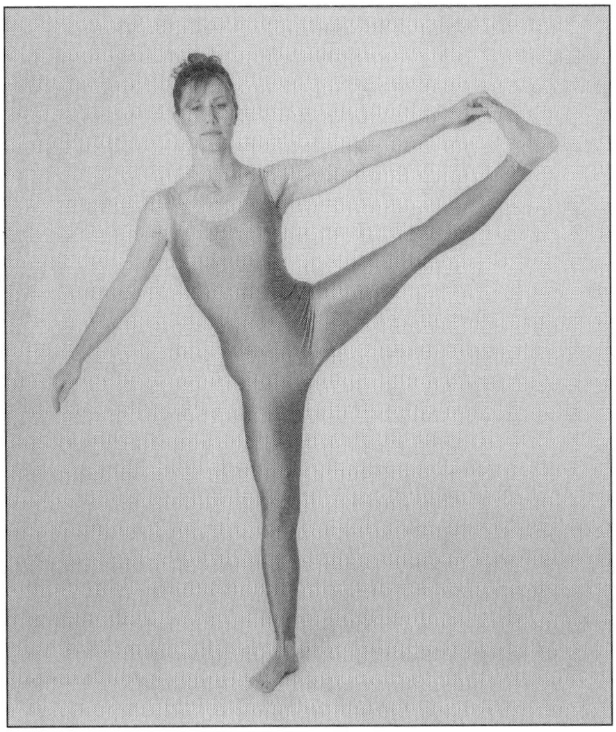

**Figure 17-13**
*Slowly swing your left leg out to the side.*

# Eagle Pose (*Garudasana*)

**Note**

*If the full extension of this posture causes too much strain on the knee, balance your toe on the floor or cross your legs and place your feet flat on the floor.*

Combined with the element of balance, the Eagle Pose gives a wonderful stretch in your upper back and shoulder area. Begin this posture by doing the arms only at first so you don't miss out on this wonderful stretch. The full extension of this posture strengthens your leg muscles while toning your upper back. It also works your hip, knee, and ankle joints while you learn to clear the mind and stay focused in order to develop balance and concentration.

1. Come into a standing position. Fix your eyes on a spot directly ahead of you. Cross your left arm over your right arm, bending them at the elbows and wrapping them around each other until the palms of your hands meet. Feel the stretch in the middle of your back. (See Figure 17-14.)

2. Bend your right knee and lower as you begin to wrap your left leg over your right leg. Continue to wrap your leg around until your foot is wrapped around the back of your right calf/ankle. Keep your heel and big toe of the standing leg down. Extend your waist upward while bending the right leg down. Do not let your knee turn outward. (See Figure 17-15.) Hold for 10 breaths as you continue to gaze at your fixed spot for balance. Concentrate on your balance.

3. Release your arms and legs and come back into a standing position with your arms resting at your sides. Rest for a few breaths.

4. Repeat with the opposite legs.

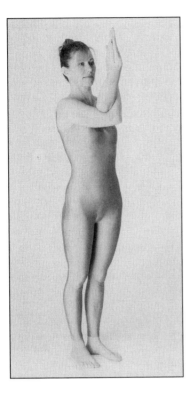

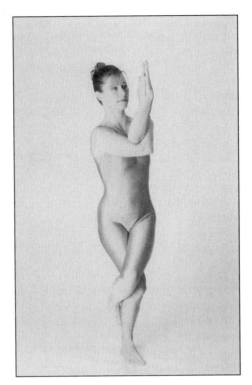

**Figure 17-14**

*Feel the stretch in the middle of your back as you wrap your arms over one another.*

**Figure 17-15**

*Bend your right knee as you lower it and wrap your left leg over your right leg. Take this slow. Feel your calf and thigh being worked and strengthened.*

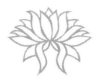

Chapter 18

# Chakra Seven

Pause and focus inward once again. Perform this brief meditation below to help activate the energy of your seventh chakra. Become aware of the emotional meaning attached to this chakra. There are no postures for your seventh chakra. Continue to open and balance your seventh chakra by going through this meditation.

*You now move up into your seventh energy center, your Crown chakra, where you begin to see a violet purple swirling at the top of your head. Your Crown chakra is your connection to God, to spirit and to your higher self. Feel the energy of the violet purple as you affirm to yourself, "I am a being of pure light and love."*

*Your Crown chakra is shaped like a funnel at the top of your head. Visualize it opening, simply by asking it to open and it will. Look up further and see your soul star above your Crown chakra. Knowledge comes from your soul star. Feel its energy as you become an open channel, attracting this energy in the form of a purple light, down into the rest of your chakras, forming a direct communication between your higher spirit and your self.*

*There are no postures for your Crown chakra. Allow the purifying energy of the purple light wash over your entire body. Feel the energy. Now that all your chakras are open and shining with the colors of the rainbow, their colors resonate the color white. Imagine your entire body filling with this white light, allowing your inner light to shine brightly.*

*As you breathe, feel yourself relaxing as you prepare for the Closing Meditation.* (See chapter 5.)

Chapter 19

# Yoga Programs

Now that you have reviewed all the postures, it may seem a little overwhelming as to where or how you should begin. To help you get started, I have included the following suggested programs to follow. Feel free to personalize your program at any time, as you become more familiar with the postures and in tune to which ones your body needs.

I have not included any relaxation, breathing or warm up exercises but it is always important to allow 5–10 minutes at the beginning of your program for these exercises, as well as some time at the end for relaxation. It is up to you to decide how much time you need to allow yourself for these important exercises. Some days will allow you more time than others.

I recommend that you do each posture three times. The first time you enter the posture is strictly for your physical body, focusing on positioning yourself safely and properly while discovering how far your body will comfortably allow you to stretch into the posture. Adjust your positioning if necessary if there is any discomfort. The second time you enter the posture, you are able to hold the stretch a little longer and see how you respond both emotionally and physically to the positioning. You are sending a message to your body as to what is required of it in order to perform this particular posture. Your body responds by limbering up the necessary body parts in order to allow you to stretch further into the posture. The third time into the posture is the most beneficial for you. Your body has received the message as to what is expected of it. You easily flow into the posture without hesitation or difficulty. Your muscles and body parts know what they are to do. There is no fear of injuring yourself at this point. You can now completely let yourself "go," experiencing the beauty and gentleness of the posture. Allow yourself to go inward and listen to how you are responding. The body/mind integration is happening and it is now that you may feel blocks, in the form of emotional energy, being released.

Remember to breathe into the postures in order to help relax the muscles involved, allowing you to enjoy and receive the benefits expected.

If you do not want to do some postures three times, please ensure that you take the time to position yourself properly and hold the posture long enough in order to gain the most benefit from it. Breathe into the stretch and hold this position until you feel your muscles loosening up and relaxing into the stretch.

All the programs outlined follow a free flow of postures.

## 20-Minute Program

1. Seated Forward Bend Series—once *(pages 109–115)*
2. Butterfly Pose *(pages 137–139)*
3. Locust *(pages 121–123)*
4. Sitting Chest Opener *(pages 201–203)*
5. Seated Spinal Twist *(pages 75–78)*
6. Camel Posture *(pages 206–209)*
7. Inverted Dog Posture *(pages 84–85)*

8. Cobra *(pages 191–192)*

9. Shoulder Stand Series *(pages 220–227)*

10. Knee Down Twist *(pages 62–63)*

## 30-Minute Program

1. Standing Chest Opener *(pages 198–200)*

2. Basic Triangle *(pages 148–149)*

3. Standing Spinal Twist *(pages 79–80)*

4. Elephant Posture—standing to seated position *(pages 128–130)*

5. Extended Leg Pose *(pages 134–136)*

6. Hip Tendon Stretch *(pages 140–142)*

7. Fish Posture *(pages 187–190)*

8. Cobra *(pages 191–192)*

9. Bow Pose *(pages 176–177)*

10. Alternate Table, Cat, Dog/Threading the Needle *(pages 81–83)*

11. Cow-Head Pose *(pages 210–211)*

12. Neck Rolls *(pages 228–230)*

## 45-Minute Program #1

1. Staff Pose *(pages 107–108)*

2. Seated Forward Bend Series—once *(pages 109–115)*

3. Hip Tendon Stretch *(pages 140–142)*

4. Butterfly Pose *(pages 137–139)*

5. Elephant Posture—seated to standing position *(pages 124–127)*

6. Extended Triangle Pose *(pages 150–151)*

7. Mountain Posture *(pages 195–197)*

8. Tree Pose *(pages 233–235)*

9. Warrior Pose *(pages 178–183)*

10. Elephant Posture—standing to seated position
    (*pages 128–130*)

11. Abdominal Strengthening Series (*pages 165–172*)

12. Knee to Chest Posture (*page 60*)

13. Locust—variation (*pages 121–122*)

14. Cobra (*pages 191–192*)

15. Inverted Dog Posture (*pages 84–85*)

16. Camel Posture (*pages 206–109*)

17. Shoulder Stand Series (*pages 220–227*)

18. Knee Down Twist (*pages 62–63*)

## 45-Minute Program #2

1. Standing Chest Opener (*pages 198–200*)

2. Basic Triangle (*pages 148–149*)

3. Extended Side Angle Pose (*pages 152–154*)

4. Standing Bow (*pages 236–238*)

5. Dancer's Pose Balancing Posture (*pages 239–243*)

6. Wrist Circles to Mountain—once
    (*pages 204–205, 195–197*)

7. Elephant Posture—standing to seated position
    (*pages 128–130*)

8. Butterfly Pose (*pages 137–139*)

9. Cobra (*pages 191–192*)

10. Lying Spinal Release (*pages 92–93*)

11. Rabbit Posture (*pages 218–219*)

12. Seated Spinal Twist (*pages 75–78*)

13. Seated Side Stretch (*pages 158–159*)

14. Abdominal Strengthening Series (*pages 165–172*)

15. Bow Pose (*pages 176–177*)

16. Camel Posture (*pages 206–209*)

17. Shoulder Stand Series (*pages 220–227*)

18. Knee Down Twist (*pages 62–63*)

Part 3

# LEARNING
# THE CHAKRAS

Chapter 20

# What Are
# the Chakras?

Although the main focus of this book is to demonstrate the postures, a very important part is to help you discover and understand your connection to your emotions, and how this connection is related to your mental and physical well-being. This is where the chakras come in. The purpose of this section is to give you a greater understanding of what the chakras mean so that you receive more benefit from your yoga program. When you have a clearer understanding of what each chakra represents, you are able to focus your attention to the areas of your body that need to be strengthened, emotionally, mentally, physically, and spiritually.

I have separated the chakras by chapter so that they can be easily referenced. Each chapter focuses on what the chakra is about and the lessons we have to learn from it. I attempt to explain each chakra in detail, beginning with its location and color. For added interest, I include a list of the glands and organs that correspond to each chakra, as well as its function and malfunction. It is interesting to see how the malfunction of a chakra can manifest itself as a physical ailment. This information makes the concept of being "linked" to your emotional body more obvious and is another source to recognizing or interpreting which of your chakras require further strengthening.

## What Is a Chakra?

Energy is the source to your "being," your physical, mental, emotional, and spiritual "being." In yoga, it is believed that your physical body is used as a vehicle to store your energy and your soul. It is for this reason, in yoga, that postures are used—to maintain a healthy physical body while activating the energy within. There are channels of energy that make up what is known as your "subtle" body, or your emotional body. We refer to these energy centers as chakras. It is the chakras that store your emotions, thoughts, and feelings, connecting your subtle body to your physical body. Activating these energy centers activates your body on all its many levels—physically, mentally, and emotionally. Looking at your emotions, thoughts, and feelings can reveal issues stored in your body, giving you the information needed to take charge of your life, promote inner healing, and better, all-round health.

Translated from Sanskrit, chakras are known as "wheels" of energy that surround the spine as they rotate around it. They are located at various places along your spine inside an invisible energy line that runs from your tailbone all the way up to the top of your head. There are seven major chakras in your body. Connected to these major energy centers are hundreds of alternate channels, called *nadis*, that play a lesser role than the major chakras, and act as a network of energy channels throughout the body connecting the major channels to all areas of the body. It is the seven major chakras that I work with in chakra yoga.

At the most basic level, our mind, emotions, and feelings are interrelated and, as explained, it is our chakras that connect them to our physical body. Each chakra is associated with its own color, energy type, personality traits, and emotional and physical functions. It is my belief that your emotions can affect your physical health. A blockage on an emotional level, such as unreleased anger, resentment, criticism, hurt feelings, guilt, or fear, creates a feeling of discomfort or "dis-ease" in the body, which in turn can create a blockage, and possibly disease, on a physical level. I was first introduced to the concept that our emotions are connected to our physical well-being from the book *You Can Heal Your Life* by Louise Hay. Now this truth has become a powerful tool in how I view my body and how I choose to heal myself and my family. Louise Hay believes that changes in your physical body can affect your body's energy system, which can affect your emotional body. As you learn to open, clear, and balance your chakras, watch where your resistance is physically, go to that chakra and learn what is holding you back emotionally. Simply put, when you are having problems or discomfort in your physical body, look to your emotions, your emotional body, to see what is going on and to learn what lessons you need to work on. Opening and balancing your chakras alongside yoga allows you to do this. You come face to face with your weaknesses and the lessons you have to learn with being your human self. You are encouraged to go within to discover your "self" and "who you are." You learn to watch how you respond to yoga on a physical, emotional, and mental level, learning and continuing to grow along the way, discovering your spirit.

It is the chakras that store prana, your energy or life force. Through chakra yoga, you can activate prana by practicing postures and breathing exercises. This stimulates them to open and release energy. Your chakras are energy centers of color, each one vibrating a color of its own. Meditating on your chakras and visualizing their corresponding colors is another way to open and activate their energy. Chakra work begins once you have relaxed your body and mind, and have entered meditation. This is achieved by doing any of the breathing and relaxation exercises outlined in part 1 and then doing the full Chakra Meditation listed in chapter 5. This meditation will not only help you become familiar with the chakras, but it will also give you an idea as to how to go into a meditation. Always remember to relax your body and to calm, or still, your mind. If you find you have a lot of "chatter" going on in your mind, ask your mind to "be still." Acknowledge the chatter as being important and that you will attend to it at a later time.

## Opening, Activating, and Balancing Your Chakras

I open each chakra chapter that follows with an affirmation that corresponds to the chakra. Saying this affirmation to yourself helps to activate the energy of the particular chakra. When you want to work on a chakra, you need to open it first. The easiest way to do this is to visualize its color and to use the affirmation to help activate the energy within. Spend a few

**Figure 20-1**

*There are seven major chakras in your body. These "wheels" of energy are located along your spine inside an invisible energy line that runs from your tailbone all the way up to the top of your head.*

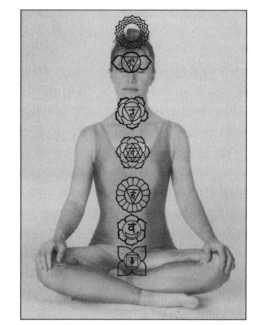

minutes concentrating on the color and trying to visualize it as a band of vibrating energy rotating in a clockwise direction, surrounding the spine. Remember to visualize the color in the back of the spine as well as the front. We often tend to visualize the color in the front only, leaving the back closed. You can not work on a chakra fully without opening the back as well. Imagine yourself breathing in the color to help you open the chakra and then focus your breath on the chakra. Try to feel the quality of the affirmation to help you activate its energy. When you can do this, you have "activated" the chakra. If you feel you need extra help in opening the chakra, ask the chakra to open. Imagine it opening and it will. Feel it opening. Use your breath to help you feel the energy swirling within.

You may not be able to see the color right away, and that is fine. Do not let this stop you. It sometimes takes months before you can actually see the colors of the chakras. It is more important to be able to "feel" the color and the quality of what the chakra represents. Be gentle on yourself and the ability to "see" will come. It may help you to visualize an object of that color to help you get started into seeing the color. For example, visualize a ruby to see the red of your first chakra, visualize an orange to see the orange of the second chakra, visualize the sun to see the yellow of the third chakra, and so on. If you see a color other than the one associated with the chakra you are opening, go with that color and with the information your mind is sending you. The color you are seeing may be used as a healing color and is the color your body can use at this time.

You may begin to see the chakra color only as a pinhole of color, or you may see black holes within the area of color you see. All of this is okay. Once again, work with what you see. A pinhole of color represents a tiny opening in that chakra and means this chakra requires some work to open it further. The blackness represents the closed state of your chakra that needs to be opened. Or, it could represent blockages in the chakra that need to be removed, dissolved, or released. This is your start, and you work from here. Work on one area of blackness at a time, asking it what it represents. Try to feel the quality of what it represents. Sit and wait for the answer. Acknowledge whatever pops into your head. It may seem insignificant or completely unrelated to what you are working on but it most likely is not. Open your mind and let the answers come. You will find a connection. This is what it means to "balance" your chakra. If it feels scary at this point, don't push yourself, however, know that getting passed this point will help you to release something that is not serving your highest good. Take your time and continue to relax yourself using your breath.

This is how you open, activate, and balance your chakras. It is important for you to balance daily as events occur that can create negative energy to settle inside you. As well, it is easy to get stuck in old thought patterns and belief systems that often prevent you from learning and growing. Balancing daily helps you to become "unstuck."

The beauty in chakra yoga lies in the ability to effectively loosen blockages by using postures alongside chakra work. Remember that your chakras are connected to your physical body. The very nature of exerting your body physically will help you to loosen yourself emotionally. It is simply another vehicle you have available to help you release. If you feel an emotion rising when doing your postures, know it is an emotional block you are releasing in that chakra. Acknowledge the emotion, then let it go.

## Releasing Blockages and Healing Your Chakras

You must go above a chakra, up to the next higher one, in order to heal the one below. All of your chakras are connected to each other in much the same way your physical body is connected by your muscles, tendons, and bones. When you want to open a chakra to release a block and heal the chakra, you need to open the chakra above it and experience the quality of that higher chakra. Using the energy and the qualities of the chakra above is your channel to releasing and healing a blockage in the chakra on which you are working. Use the energy of the higher chakra to understand what it is you need to work on and what you should do to get there. For instance, when you feel a strong emotion such as anger, it is felt in your third chakra. You need to express those feelings to prevent them from settling in your body. You use your fifth chakra, the Throat, to express your feelings. However, you must pass through your fourth chakra, the one directly above the third, in order to release the emotional feelings properly and completely. The fourth chakra is your Heart chakra. Use the qualities of the Heart chakra—compassion, empathy, forgiveness, and discernment—as you express what it is you need to release. Do not bypass your Heart chakra and express yourself by hurting or disempowering the next person. When you have released by using the qualities of the chakra above, do not worry about how the next person reacts. Using the example above, if you have come from your Heart and expressed yourself without laying blame on the other person, you have done what is best for you. If the other person reacts negatively, this is because they have their own issues to deal with.

Your emotional body plays an integral role as to how your body functions and how you respond to your environment. Pay attention to your feelings and emotions and to "how" they are making your physical body "feel." Make the connection. "Feel" the connection. It is there. Pay attention to your body and how you feel. As you discover your connection to your emotional body you become more conscious to the lessons you need to learn and to how you choose to live. In this way you are able to learn your human lessons and grow as you continue on your journey of self-discovery and find your way to developing a more healthy and balanced approach to your life.

It is my hope that this section will give you an understanding of the chakras, and what each one represents. As I work with my chakras, I learn more and more of their meaning and what they represent. (One of the more informative books I have come across on the subject of chakras is a book by Anodea Judith titled *Wheels of Life: A User's Guide to the Chakra System [Llewellyn, 1987].*)

Chapter 21

# All About
# Chakra One

*"I am safe and secure."*

The first chakra is also referred to as your Root chakra.
It vibrates out from the very base of your spine, your
tailbone, glowing a deep ruby red energy. This is a stabilizing, grounding energy, helping you to feel at peace
with yourself and full of confidence. When your first
chakra is balanced and functioning properly, it's energy
firmly roots you to Mother Earth. You are full of physical energy and enjoy being physically active. You are
comfortable with who you are and enjoy being with and
around other people.

The element associated with the first chakra is earth.
As we become rooted to earth through this chakra, her
grounding energy helps you become stronger and more
secure with who you are. You feel safe and secure, fully
grounded, stabilized and nurtured by the energy of
Mother Earth, helping you to feel comfortable in your

**Figure 21-1**

*The first chakra is your Root chakra. It vibrates out from the very base of your spine, your tailbone. This is a stabilizing, grounding energy, helping you to feel at peace with yourself and full of confidence.*

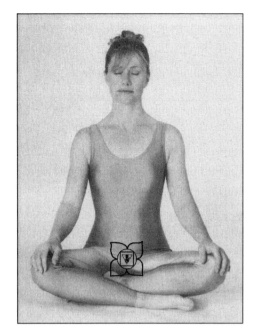

body. The first chakra is the most stable of the chakras and it is from this foundation that all the other chakras are supported. As you look at all your chakras and strive to experience what it means to be fully human, it is necessary for you to experience the energies of all the chakras. This cannot be done unless the chakras are worked on equally. This was best captured for me in an article I read several years ago on chakra meditation, by Pat Ohlendorf-Moffat, in which it was explained in order to have a complete human experience, we need to experience both the denser, more physical energies of the lower chakras as well as the lighter, more spiritual and emotional energies of the higher chakras. This statement will become clearer to you as you gain a more thorough understanding of the chakras.

The first chakra deals with your ability to survive and all the basic necessities you need for physical survival. Any issues revolving around food, shelter, or money is a first chakra issue. It is here that our primal instinct to survive is put into action. It is not until these basic necessities

## Chakra One Table[1]

**Location:** Base of spine at the tailbone

**Color:** Red, ruby red

**Gland:** Adrenals[2]

**Organs:** Large intestine meridian
Muscles

**Body parts:** Hips, legs, knees, feet, ankles
Spine, especially the lower back
Blood
Immune system

**Function:** Survival, security
Confidence
Generosity
Grounding
Breaking away from societal beliefs

**Malfunction:** Leg problems, knee troubles, varicose veins, sciatica
Spinal problems such as back pain, scoliosis
Hemorrhoids
Obesity
Anorexia nervosa
Degenerative arthritis
Cancers (can begin here from unexpressed emotions)
Constipation/diarrhea
Fibromyalgia
Chronic fatigue syndrome
Skin problems
Auto-immune diseases
Materialistic greed

are looked after that we are able to move on to developing ourselves fully as human beings.

Misuse of the basic survival necessities is a sign that you are stuck in an unbalanced Root chakra. Chronic aches and pains, eating disorders, and financial worries are an indication that your first chakra is obstructed. You may tend to be unhappy, cruel, or overimpulsive, or have the feeling of being out of touch with yourself or with those around you.

Your adrenal gland is the gland involved with your first chakra. It is the adrenals that cause you to operate from a "fight or flight" instinct when in an uncomfortable situation. When you operate from this instinct, you cage yourself in, back to those restrictions you placed yourself in. Learn to break down those barriers so that you can see other perspectives and the different ways to react to a situation. The first chakra deals with living within the restrictions we tend to place on ourselves, and how we learn to step outside those restrictions to take risks. As you step outside you are taught to look at other perspectives in life, to pause instead of reacting to a situation.

Although the first chakra's focus is primarily on physical survival, it also relates to emotional survival. It is here that your feelings and attitudes about society, religion, family, and friends are registered and implanted into your consciousness. You grow up with these feelings, feelings not only from childhood but from all your relationships including marriage, and this is how your own belief systems are formed. Emotional fear is registered here as well, your self-image and/or the image you feel you do not live up to.

The back and/or spine is what supports your body. Louise Hay explains in her book *You Can Heal Your Life* that problems with your back can represent feelings of not being supported. Problems in different areas of your back represent different things. Lower back problems are a result of an imbalance in your first chakra and can be related to basic survival issues, such as one revolving around money. Problems in other areas of the back are discussed in chakra three and four, as they relate to these chakras and/or body areas.

Meditating on this chakra, as I explained at the beginning of this section, will help to balance all your chakras as it is the first chakra that supports all the rest. Keeping your first chakra open and free of obstruction sets the tone to balancing all your chakras. As always, remember to open the back of the chakra while opening the front. As mentioned above, lower back problems can be a result of an issue with a basic survival issue (i.e., money). Getting to the root of your issues and allowing them to be released can prevent the back problem from manifesting.

Know judgment when in meditation; be gentle and patient with yourself. If you have trouble opening a chakra, allow yourself time to allow it to open, when it is ready, never pushing yourself. You may not be ready to face an issue at this time. Choose your own rate of growth or acceleration. Society's rate of growth, as a whole, is very slow.

## Lessons from Chakra One

### *Belief Systems*

What you learn from the first chakra is to express your feelings, and to release the feelings or ideas that no longer nourish you, or serve your higher purpose. Acknowledge the feelings as once having served a purpose. Now that you've grown, they are no longer needed. Thank them and let them go. If you have trouble letting the feelings go, try visualizing yourself placing them inside a balloon. When you have placed all your negative feelings inside the balloon, let the balloon go. Watch it fly away, and symbolically with it, your negative feelings.

If you feel that someone or something has let you down, look to your own belief systems to see if they need changing. Cancers in the physical body are from unexpressed feelings in the emotional body, explains Louise Hay, feelings of hatred and resentment. Take responsibility for your own beliefs, and feel confident to break away from them if they no longer serve your higher purpose. Create your own reality. Watch opposing beliefs and let them go if need be. The first chakra teaches you to not take in other people's beliefs as your own reality but rather to stand firm in your own beliefs.

### *Look at Other Perspectives*

As your first chakra develops and grows stronger, you become more comfortable with who you are and the belief systems you support as your own. You learn to have the courage to step outside the walls you place around yourself for protection, and to step into that unfamiliar place for testing. It is okay to feel a little uneasy with these new surroundings. Having the courage to test the new ground instead of running away from it is how you learn to grow. Baby steps forward are better than no steps at all.

## Notes

1. Dr. Fedor Zelina, naturopath; Fazia Khan, certified yoga instructor, lecture notes, 1996–1997; Anodea Judith, *Wheels of Life: A User's Guide to the Chakra System* (Llewellyn Publications, 1987); Christiane Northrup, M.D., *Women's Bodies, Women's Wisdom* (Bantam Books, 1994).

2. Adrenals govern the function of the kidneys and are responsible for the immune system of the body, the effects of infection and stress on the body, and the regulation of sugar metabolism. The adrenals also produce DHEA, the mother hormone.

Chapter 22

# All About Chakra Two

*"I create with love."*

The second chakra is also known as your Sacral chakra. The powerful light from this chakra vibrates out from the center of your pelvis, about 2 inches below the navel. The energy glows a vibrant deep-orange or red-orange color, covering your entire lower abdomen area including your hips, womb, and genitals. The Sacral chakra is the center of your sexual and creative energy, your passions and desires. In her article on chakra meditations, Pat Ohlendorf-Moffat describes this energy as the kind of energy that attracts you to the opposite sex. It is also the kind of energy that attracts you to the things you love to do.

The element this chakra is associated with is water. It follows that the second chakra has to do with all the "watery" elements of the body—menstrual flow, seminal fluid, urine, and fluid in the intestines, as well as circulation. Water symbolizes continuous movement and the

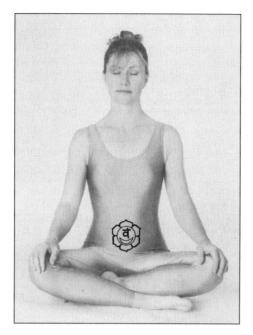

**Figure 21-1**

*The second chakra is also known as your Sacral chakra. It is located at the center of your pelvis, about 2 inches below the navel. It is the center of your sexual and creative energy, your passions and desires.*

freedom we need in order to create. We are continually changing as we grow and learn.

The second chakra has to do with your relationship to others and how you relate to them on a "one-to-one" basis. It also has to do with creativity and your emotions. The second chakra's focus is on your earliest and most basic emotions, your sense of belonging to your family or a group, your feelings of being accepted and/or worthy. When your second chakra is balanced, you have a healthy sense of emotional security and of "who you are." Your sense of belonging is strong and secure. You have a cheerful, friendly, and positive temperament and are not afraid to express how you feel. As well, you are sensitive to the needs of others. An unbalanced Sacral chakra leads to difficulty getting in touch with your own feelings. You may be uncomfortable when around others or be overly sensitive to comments made to you or about you. You may tend to have a bad temper or to hold in your emotions and them blow up over a small issue. You may have issues over money, tend to be competitive, or feel the need to defend yourself, either physically or emotionally. It is in your second chakra that creative "abortion" can

## *Chakra Two Table*[1]

Location: Center of the pelvis, 2 inches below the navel

Color: Orange to red-orange

Gland: Ovaries and testicles, the glands involved in creating life; they also govern hormonal activity in the body

Organs: Kidneys: absorb and detoxify fear

Spleen: houses and processes worry

Body Parts: Hips, uterus, womb, genitals

Appendix

Bladder

Function: Desire and pleasure

Sexuality and procreation

Relationship to others on an emotional level

Malfunction: Ovary/prostrate problems

Uterine, bladder, or kidney trouble

Pelvis/lower back pain

High blood pressure

Diabetes

Appendicitis and pancreatic ailments

Paranoia

Impotence/frigidity

Incest/sexual abuse

happen—that is, where creative ideas stop, usually out of fear (i. e., money issues, competition, or feelings of unworthiness).

## Lessons from Chakra Two

### *Creative Center*

The Sacral chakra is about sexual and creative energy. In order to be creative, you need to express yourself freely and openly, without fear. When you can do this, you feel a sense of fullness or abundance. You learn that you create from love because life was created from love. Our basic understanding is to come from love. If you find you are having a struggle with something or someone, ask yourself, "Am I doing this with love?" Pay attention to what your answer is, and watch what happens. If you change your actions to those coming from love you may notice the struggle begins to dissipate and the actions needed to overcome the difficulty become more clear.

### *Recognize Your Feelings and Emotions*

Your second chakra also deals with your relationship with others and how you feel about them. Your feelings have to do with how you feel internally. It is a "state of being"; for example, "I feel hurt." Your emotions are energy in motion, expressing your feelings externally, for example, anger, happiness, sadness. What you learn from being in your second chakra is to express your feelings before they start brewing, and to express emotions as emotions. It is often seen as inappropriate for adults or older children to express or communicate emotionally so they may tend to "bank" their feelings of anger, resulting in inappropriate blow-ups. They blow up and then feel guilty. It is important to express emotions as they occur, and to express them in an appropriate manner. When negative feelings are left to settle in your body, they can begin to cause discomfort or "dis-ease" in the body. As I explained at the beginning of chapter 20 about what the chakras are, you must go to the chakra above to heal the chakra below. In this case, go up to your third chakra to feel what emotion you're feeling. Continue going up through your fourth chakra to allow yourself to come from your Heart chakra, and then express what you're feeling through your fifth chakra, which is your Throat chakra.

Learn to recognize and respect the emotions you feel in your second chakra. Be aware that you can pick up on other people's feelings, and that you may need to distinguish between your feelings and theirs. It is not damaging to pick up on other people's happiness. But the negative energy from other people can pull you down and lower your energy. It is draining, and can be damaging if you are constantly being drawn into other people's negativity. Watch your energy field's vitality if you think you are still plugged into another person or even your past. You need to be aware of who you are "plugged" into, being careful not to get drawn into negative energy, such as fear, depression, or even violence.

## *Trust*

Your second chakra also teaches you to trust. Trust is at the opposite end of fear. If you find you can not trust others, look within to find out where your fear is coming. You must first learn to trust yourself, your thoughts and actions before you can trust others. On the surface trust relates to your ability to deal with others, however, this cannot happen sincerely or honestly until you are honest with yourself, being honest with your feelings of security and of "who you are."

To trust others, trust who you are. Trust your actions and responses as being appropriate, as well as your emotions and feelings. Have trust in yourself and the things in your life that make you feel good about yourself. Trust involves opening your heart and letting go of the fear. Feel your feelings and accept them as being a part of who you are. It is not until you can trust your feelings and who you are that you can go beyond this, and learn to trust others. Do not worry if you can not yet trust others. It will come. The more you learn to trust yourself and your feelings, the closer you will become to trusting others. It can be said that as you grow to be more trusting, the more trustworthy you become as a person.

## Notes

1. Dr. Fedor Zelina, naturopath; Fazia Khan, certified yoga instructor, lecture notes, 1996–1997; Anodea Judith, *Wheels of Life: A User's Guide to the Chakra System* (Llewellyn Publications, 1987); Christiane Northrup, M.D., *Women's Bodies, Women's Wisdom* (Bantam Books, 1994).

Chapter 23

# All About Chakra Three

*"I feel my feelings."*

The third chakra glows a powerful golden sunshine yellow and is located between the base of your rib cage and approximately 2 inches above your navel, including the stomach. Understanding that our emotional/mental body is linked to our physical body, as explained by Louise Hay in her book *You Can Heal Your Life*, it follows that the function of the third chakra is often compared to the function of the stomach, the place we "digest" new ideas and experiences. (As we know, the primary function of the stomach is to digest foods consumed into our physical body. Likewise, on an emotional level, the stomach is where our ability to "digest" new ideas, experiences, or beliefs is exercised. )

The third chakra is known as the Solar Plexus chakra, but is also referred to as your Power center, your Action center, or your Emotional center. This is where the pow-

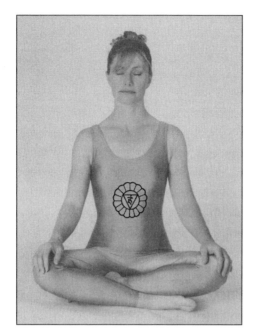

**Figure 23-1**

*The third chakra is known as the Solar Plexus chakra. It is located between the base of your rib cage and approximately 2 inches above your navel. This is where the powerful energy of your emotions and feelings reside.*

erful energy of your emotions and feelings reside, and where you act on those feelings. It is also where you house your personal power and your own personal energy, which manifests itself in the form of your emotions and feelings as they relate to your personality. Shock and stressful events affect this chakra, even the sort of daily stress caused from trying to handle too many situations in a day without taking some time out for relaxation. If you are depleted of energy after a stressful situation, know you are operating from a "bare bones" capacity. Take a few minutes to center yourself, to recharge yourself, so to speak. Acknowledge the messages from your body.

The energy of this chakra is strong and powerful, an energy that connects you to the people around you. This is where you develop a sense of personal power as a member of your community as well as with your family and friends. How you relate to others and the sense of satisfaction you get from these relationships will determine how you feel about yourself, your self-image.

The Solar Plexus chakra also deals with the relationship you have with yourself and whether or not you see yourself as worthy. This is

# Chakra Three Table[1]

| | |
|---|---|
| **Location:** | Two inches above the navel, between the base of the rib cage and the navel; the abdominal area |
| **Color:** | Golden sunshine yellow |
| **Gland:** | Pancreas<br>Adrenals |
| **Organs:** | Liver<br>Spleen<br>Duodenum<br>Gallbladder |
| **Body Parts:** | Abdomen/stomach<br>Middle of the back<br>Upper intestines<br>Lower esophagus |
| **Function:** | Will<br>Power: use of personal power and emotions<br>Relationship to self: self-esteem, self-confidence, self-respect |
| **Malfunction:** | Ulcers<br>Diabetes: an extension from the second chakra<br>Hypoglycemia<br>Anger<br>Colon/intestinal problems, colitis, irritable bowel syndrome<br>Indigestion, stomach problems<br>Gallstones<br>Anorexia/bulimia<br>Hepatitis<br>Feelings of inferiority |

where you register your feelings about your self-image, and the approval or criticism of yourself. It is where you experience the action of breaking away from "the tribe," from societal beliefs. This is where you let go of attachments and feel comfortable with yourself for doing so. It is a difficult chakra to master, and many people give up here. It is easier to convince yourself that things are okay or to go along with what others believe because standing your own ground and breaking away from what others believe causes too much discomfort and turmoil. The discomfort is felt in your stomach, this discomfort stemming from your fear of change or making a mistake, or perhaps your fear of letting others down. Realize that fear is useful when viewed as a signal that something in your life requires attention. It can then be used as an opportunity for growth. An old belief system or pattern needs to be released and this is your opportunity to change. When you are able to successfully break away from old beliefs, there is a birthing of a new you. Try and see the positives in your life. Use fear in a positive way instead of only seeing it's destructive values.

Your third chakra is where such questions as "Who am I?" are asked. You have confidence in your opinion and the decisions you make and do not feel the need to push them onto other people. You do not feel left out or uncomfortable in groups and are able to join into conversation without feeling the need to dominate, showing respect for yourself as well as for others. It is from the third chakra that you develop a strong sense of loyalty to friendships, creating a sense of satisfaction in yourself.

The element associated with the third chakra is fire, the flame of burning energy or substances representing the burning nature of our emotions. Fire is a powerful and growing force fueled by energy, confident on one end of the spectrum, destructive on the other. The third chakra is where you carry your anger, hostility, and the feeling of being threatened. But, this is also where you are able learn courage and develop strength to overcome these negative emotions. It is your "clearing house" of emotions, as you symbolically use the fire to clear these emotions. While it can be used to clear your body of negative emotions, making room for new, positive ones, fire can also be destructive. Your feelings can become inflamed and ignite quickly into something dangerous. If attended to, negative feelings can easily be blown out.

When left alone to burn, they can grow out of control, taking on a life of their own. Fire is also used to represent the ardent or zealous nature of your emotions—the burning passion or the intense feelings of desire you may have for another or for a cause.

The third chakra is the center of your psychic body. It is important to know that "knowing" your psychic body is restricted to only the experiences of the soul and therefore to the validity of your feelings. You "feel" the truth and what is good and bad. You can also take in other people's thoughts through your Solar Plexus. This, too, may affect the validity of your truth. Remember to guard yourself, if necessary, from other people's thoughts. You can do this simply by covering your tummy with your hand to act as a barrier. Or, when in meditation, visualize yourself being wrapped in a cocoon of blue light. The blue light is a protective light and will serve to block out negative feelings entering your aura. Do this visualization during your daily meditation, especially if you know you will be in an environment of negativity that day. You can also cocoon your family and loved ones if they are affected by other's negative feelings. The covering will protect you from any negative thoughts or feelings entering your aura.

When your third chakra is strong and well developed, you will have respect for yourself and you will be able to control your emotions. You will enjoy being physically active because a strong third chakra lends to plenty of physical strength and endurance. When your third chakra is operating properly, the effect of adrenaline produced by the adrenals is not uncomfortable to the body. When you live in a balanced third chakra, you tend to have a love for nature and the elements.

As discussed earlier, your Solar Plexus chakra is where you house your emotions, including your negative feelings. Because of this, when you are weak in this chakra, you may have difficulty making decisions and have a sense of inadequacy about yourself. You may feel people are out to get you or that you are not strong enough to speak up, denying your own best interests in order to please others. You may become overcompetitive and/or jealous. It is here that we experience blaming, i.e., blaming our parents, spouses, or friends for not living up to our own expectations. Know that souls come together for healing, to allow healing to happen. We choose to come together as a family for healing.

Problems in the middle of your back, where your third chakra is, can stem from feelings of guilt or fear from not looking at what we are hiding from ourselves, explains Louise Hay. We throw our issues behind us instead of dealing with them.

## Lessons from Chakra Three
### *Dealing with your Emotions and Feelings*

The third chakra has to do with how you handle situations, and your feelings or emotions that arise from these situations. Are you comfortable or uncomfortable? Are you "at ease" or "ill at ease," which is where the word "dis-ease," or disease, stems from. When you are feeling uncomfortable, the third chakra teaches you to go up to the fourth chakra, to the Heart chakra, instead of going down and fighting or denying the feelings that are there. Remember to go up to the next chakra in order to heal the one below. The qualities of the Heart chakra will help you follow through with your feelings in a positive and loving way, trusting yourself and your feelings as real. You have a choice. You can come from your lower energies when dealing with a situation, or you can go up to the Heart chakra, to a higher, more loving energy. Whatever your choice, do not become involved in judging yourself. Judgement has to do with the ego. It involves comparison and not wanting to look at your "self."

Do not be afraid to make mistakes in life, as long as you learn from them. Making mistakes are meant to help us learn our lessons in life. If you keep on making the same mistakes over and over again, however, then know you are not learning and listening to the messages being sent to you.

### *Honor and Respect*

Your third chakra teaches you to live with an honor code. Once you have made a decision, stick with it. Do not be swayed by other people's thoughts. Focus on your integrity, your personal honor, your ethics and self-discipline. State your boundaries and the things that are not acceptable to you. Do not feel the need to explain yourself. This chakra teaches you to learn to stand in your own power, and that when you need to stand into that area of the unknown, to do it without fear, having faith in yourself. It is from learning to stand in your own power that you learn self-respect. If you can not respect yourself, you can not give it to another.

Respect has to do with how we communicate with one another. We learn that what we want to achieve in communication is to be heard and to be acknowledged, to simply have a positive energy exchange. If you can not show empathy in communication, you have a block that needs to be removed. Do not say things if it only becomes a power issue for you. You have a choice. You can use your emotions for power, or you can use them to heal. This is why the Throat chakra is placed above the Heart chakra. We must go through the step of passing through the Heart chakra, of loving ourselves, before speaking out our emotions.

This is a difficult chakra to master. We are often weak in our Solar Plexus, our abdominal area. Remember that our emotional body is connected to our physical body. If you are weak in your physical body, you are prone to being weak on an emotional level as well. It is important to keep your third chakra strong both physically and emotionally so that when you need to handle daily situations, you can do so with ease and a sense of confidence. Women are especially prone to having weaker abdominal muscles, especially after their childbearing years, and so they are often seen as being weaker on an emotional level. The most direct way to strengthen your this chakra is by using your physical body, by strengthening your abdominal muscles. This is why I have included an assortment of abdominal postures that deal specifically with strengthening your abdominal muscles. The more abdominal strengthening exercises you do, the stronger your abdominal area becomes. The stronger you are physically, the stronger you are emotionally.

Pay attention to your thoughts. In relationships, honor each other. Compromise. Watch what you are thinking. Your thoughts count and can create action. You are held accountable. Watch your criticism and judgment as well. Learn to avoid making judgmental comments. Relationships may falter when working on this chakra because of its "fiery" nature.

Pay attention to your feelings. Listen to the messages your body is sending you. Learn to view fear in a positive manner, as a signal that something in your life is making you feel uncomfortable. Something needs to be worked on, or changed. This is an opportunity for growth.

## Notes

1. Dr. Fedor Zelina, naturopath; Fazia Khan, certified yoga instructor, lecture notes, 1996–1997; Anodea Judith, *Wheels of Life: A User's Guide to the Chakra System* (Llewellyn Publications, 1987); Christiane Northrup, M.D., *Women's Bodies, Women's Wisdom* (Bantam Books, 1994).

## Chapter 24

# All About Chakra Four

*"My heart is open."*

The fourth chakra is known as your Heart chakra. It vibrates with a clear, bright emerald green energy in the middle of the chest, out the middle of the back, between the shoulder blades and down to the arms, hands and fingers. The Heart chakra represents love, compassion, harmony, and empathy. As this energy vibrates, it attracts a loving energy, opening the chakra. With an open fourth chakra, you are happy, loving, and feel connected to the people around you. It is also your center for forgiveness. Forgiveness is not just in the mind. You feel forgiveness in the heart. Once you have forgiven, you will be tested to see if you have released the hurt feelings. When forgiveness truly comes from the heart, you learn to let go completely with no perception of betrayal.

The element associated with the fourth chakra is air. As much as air is a mixture of surrounding gases that

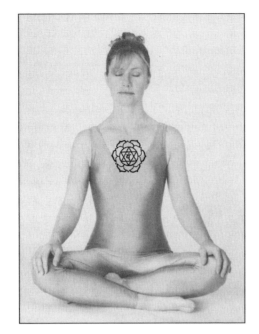

**Figure 24-1**

*The fourth chakra is known as your Heart chakra. It is located in the middle of the chest. The Heart chakra represents love, compassion, harmony, and empathy.*

form its atmosphere, so is the Heart chakra a mixture of the body's energies, forming the atmosphere of your body and the apparent character of who you are.

The Heart chakra is the communicator to the entire body, through circulation and feelings, such that the element of air becomes symbolic of circulation. The Heart chakra's key function deals with the heart and lungs, the pumping of blood through the heart and the act of breathing through the lungs. Breathing not only includes the act of inhaling and exhaling air but also the act of circulating air throughout the body. Air is essential to life, our essential life force, or prana. Without air life ceases to exist and the spirit and body separate.

The fourth chakra is where you get your confidence, because with an open heart, you feel strong. And when you are strong and your Heart chakra is open, you love life and all it has to offer. You believe that all people are equal yet here on earth for their own purpose. As well, you tend to surround yourself with a sense of calm no matter what is happening around you. The Heart chakra is where you feel your joys and sorrows, and how deeply they are felt. Because an open

# Chakra Four Table[1]

| | |
|---|---|
| **Location:** | Heart area from the base of the rib cage to the base of the throat, including the back, shoulders, arms and hands |
| **Color:** | Emerald green |
| **Gland:** | Thymus (key to the body's immune system and works with the adrenals) |
| **Organs:** | Heart (pumping of the heart for blood circulation)<br>Lungs (breathing for air circulation) |
| **Body Parts:** | Shoulders, arms, hands, fingers<br>Ribs<br>Breasts, chest<br>Upper back area<br>Diaphragm, upper esophagus |
| **Function:** | Love, harmony, and compassion<br>Forgiveness<br>Communicator to the entire body (circulation and feelings)<br>Transformer (issues are transmuted or dissolved when we come from a place in our heart, from love) |
| **Malfunction:** | Asthma<br>Lung disease and/or lung cancer<br>Heart ailments, heart disease, high blood pressure<br>Upper back/shoulder problems<br>Breast problems including cancer<br>Allergies<br>Pneumonia<br>An "emotionally" closed heart promotes envy, selfishness, unresolved issues, difficulty accepting or giving love |

Heart chakra allows you to feel strength and confidence with who you are, you are not afraid to express your emotions of happiness or sorrow, laughing or crying without fear of what others may think.

Not allowing the opportunity to enjoy life's pleasures can cause damage to your fourth chakra. A feeling of tightness in your upper back or behind your shoulder blades could represent an emotional blockage in the back of your fourth chakra. As explained before, remember to open both the front and back of a chakra when working on it so that blockages have the opportunity to be released. Problems in the upper back, which is part of the fourth chakra, may have to do with your feelings of emotional support, explains Louise Hay in her book *You Can Heal Your Life*—feelings that people do not understand or support you. Any blockage in this chakra can cause tension throughout your entire body. As your emotions become heavy, you may notice a difference in your breathing. It too may become heavy. You may tend to judge others and have an overbearing, know-it-all attitude. You may become unreliable or tend to give love only when certain conditions are met. Living your life with a constricted or closed fourth chakra perpetuates negativity, especially in stress situations. This can eventually lead to heart problems in the physical body.

The Heart chakra responds to honesty and truthfulness. The more you ask for and tell the truth, the more your this chakra will open. The fourth chakra can be damaged and begins to close by telling lies, even the little lies we sometimes tell in order to protect the feelings of others. Injury can even be caused when you accept an untruth without challenge.

## Lessons from Chakra Four

### *Discernment*

The Heart chakra teaches us "knowing." We are back in the place of our innocence as the Heart transforms our "adult" back to our "child," to our carefree and fearless self. We remember the sense of freedom we had as children, but now we are able to appreciate that freedom. The fourth chakra is where we hear the answers, but now we hear them with wisdom and discernment. The Heart chakra knows discernment, or discretion. It has to do with being aware of the energy around us and making the choice whether or not to interact with this energy. You learn to make your choices by choosing the right vibration, listening and feeling for the right answer. Discernment has to do with learning to stand back and pause before making a decision. To detach yourself from a situation which gives you the opportunity to come from your higher self. You do what is best for your higher self. The fourth chakra is the transformer or gateway between the lower and higher chakras, where transformation happens between the two. Issues are transmuted or dissolved when you come from a place in your heart, from love. The Heart chakra is the link between body and spirit.

## Love

The Heart chakra is where we experience spiritual love, that is, self-love as opposed to being selfish. It deals with spiritual joy and not material joy. It is where we experience life's pleasures and where we may ask the question "Why am I unhappy?" It is where we go to pursue our connection to spirit or God. As we pursue this spiritual connection, our expectations of personal relationships may change, from a relationship based on financial/emotional security to one of respect and honorable love.

The Heart chakra teaches us that love is not doing other's work but allowing the other person their own process, their own journey. We learn not to be angered or frustrated by another's journey. You may not agree with someone's decisions, but you are able to support them. This center teaches us forgiveness, forgiving others for being who they are and for the way they act. We recognize that we all have to deal with our own issues.

Expanding on the theory that you must go up to a higher chakra in order to heal the one below, the Heart chakra is the vehicle for expressing the emotions you feel in your third chakra. Use your Heart chakra to unlock the feelings in your physical body. When you come from your heart, you are coming from a place of fullness, without attachment of irritation or exhaustion. You realize that communication is an energy exchange and that we can empower one another with our thoughts as they are expressed, but only when we speak from the heart. Your intent, the place your messages come from, should always come from the heart, from love, from your higher consciousness. Defensive communication is not coming from the heart and it is a sign that you are not strong in your third chakra or in your knowledge. If your intention is to upset the other person or if you want them to resonate with your hurt feelings, then this is a power issue for you. It is your ego coming in. Your ego loves separation. It has a stubbornness that will not allow you to switch over to your heart. The heart, on the other hand, enjoys union. Instead of coming from your lower, denser energies, try coming from your higher, lighter ones. To learn what love is begins with learning to love yourself, qualifying your feelings, and your actions and thoughts with love and self-acceptance.

## Balance

This energy center is where you give and receive. You give and receive gifts with your hands. You exchange hugs and greetings with your hands. Remember to balance by giving and receiving—inviting the opposite energy into your energy field, into your being. When you do this there will be no struggle or resistance because you have made the choice to move toward lightness. Consciously balance who you are. Step out of your safety, your familiar place that is safe and invite the other energy in to balance.

It follows that in your Heart chakra you experience the balance of the male and female energies within each of us. The yin and yang principle, one being negative and feminine (yin), the other being positive and masculine (yang), the interaction of the two influencing the destiny of your being. As you focus on your fourth chakra, the halfway point, go within to balance the male and female energies in you. To balance, you first need to take responsibility for who you are and to understand the emotional connection you have to your male and female energies. This will depend on your ability to respond to yourself.

Following the ying-yang principle, the left side of your body represents your female energy, your nurturing, caring, devoted, or empathetic nature. It is here that you take in your feminine energy and where issues involving women and/or your mother are registered. The right side of your body represents your male energy, your outgoing, more physical, assertive, and confident nature. It is here that you take in your male energy, and where issues revolving around men and/or your father are registered. A woman needs to learn to find her identity within and to learn assertiveness, courage, and independence. A man needs to focus on nurturing, caring and empathy. It is easier for a woman to overcome barriers and balance because she can go outside of herself, to her external environment, to find solutions. Men, on the other hand, are accustomed to and comfortable with using their external environment. They have to learn to go within, to their female energy, to learn how to express their feelings and needs. It is not about being weak or aggressive, or about blaming one another. It is about acknowledging your feelings and balancing your yin and yang so that the decisions you make come from a higher conscience. Our first caregivers are our parents from whom we learn about our male/female qualities. If you have issues with either of your parents, then you may not have yet claimed that male/female part of you. You may not have yet fully accessed or experienced that part of you. You need to go within to find it.

It is in the fourth chakra that we meet in silence. The silence is not an escape or a weapon. Silence is where we find ourselves. It is where we can go to find our answers. It is a nurturing space and a meeting place of the male and female energies. Learning to quiet the mind is empowering because in this place where the mind is quiet we are able to hear the answers.

## Notes

1. Dr. Fedor Zelina, naturopath; Fazia Khan, certified yoga instructor, lecture notes, 1996–1997; Anodea Judith, *Wheels of Life: A User's Guide to the Chakra System* (Llewellyn Publications, 1987); Christiane Northrup, M.D., *Women's Bodies, Women's Wisdom* (Bantam Books, 1994).

Chapter 25

# All About Chakra Five

*"My throat is open."*

The fifth chakra is known as your Throat chakra and is located at the center of your neck. The color of this energy center shines the color of the sky—sky blue. It shines outward from your throat in the front of your body, and from the base of your neck at the back, covering your jaws, cheeks, nose, eyes, and ears, all the way up to just below the eyebrows and the back of the head as well. The sky blue energy of the Throat chakra shimmers the truth, giving you the courage to speak up and to speak the truth without blaming others. The back of your neck is where you hold your will power, the front, your emotions. This is often why you are unable to speak when under emotional stress because your emotions are blocking your throat. When opening your fifth chakra, as explained before, remember to open both the

**Figure 25-1**

*The fifth chakra is known as your Throat chakra and is located at the center of your neck. This chakra shimmers the truth, giving you the courage to speak up and to speak the truth.*

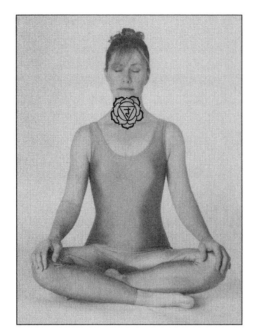

front and the back of this chakra, so that your will is exercised and your emotions are released.

The element associated with the fifth chakra is sound—sound through vibration and communication. It is through this chakra that we express ourselves to the world around us. It is your center for communicating, such as speaking and singing, and as we grow and mature, so too does this chakra. The Throat chakra is also your center for creativity and learning, as you express yourself through your learning, creating, and growing into the unique individual you see yourself as becoming. My meditation instructor and advisor, Kathy Roseborough, once told me that when someone is in a well-suited profession, their Throat chakra will blossom.

The body parts involved with your fifth chakra include your eyes, ears, nose, and mouth, and so it follows that when your Throat chakra is working well, all your senses are sharp, including your sense of touch. You think and speak clearly. You say what you mean but in a positive way so as not to offend or put people off. You are not afraid to speak up nor do you engage in verbal insult or abuse. It is from here

## Chakra Five Table[1]

| | |
|---|---|
| **Location:** | Centered in the hollow of the throat, but covers the area from the base of the throat up to the place just below the eyebrows |
| **Color:** | Sky blue |
| **Gland:** | Thyroid (regulates the metabolic function in the body) |
| | Parathyroid (regulates calcium metabolism) |
| **Organs:** | Brain |
| **Body Parts:** | Face, including the eyes (they communicate our emotions), ears, mouth, nose, chin, cheeks, teeth, and gums |
| | Throat |
| | Bronchial tubes, trachea |
| | Neck, neck vertebrae |
| **Function:** | Communication and the ability to speak out |
| | Creative expression |
| | Projection of power and creative energy |
| | Leadership |
| **Malfunction:** | Throat problems, hoarseness |
| | Neck problems |
| | Nose problems |
| | Weeping eyes (when expressing emotions) |
| | Hearing problems |
| | Teeth and gum problems |
| | Colds, bronchitis, laryngitis |
| | Thyroid problems |
| | Abusive power and control over others |
| | Inability to speak up |

that any thoughts of failure are being mastered. You begin to take responsibility for your "self" and begin to take chances.

Your Throat chakra will begin to close down if you ignore the information your senses bring in. When your fifth chakra begins to close, you will not be able to speak up or articulate your feelings or you may tend to blurt out your emotions without thinking and then feel upset about what you said. Usually, your Throat chakra closes down from not being used (not speaking up), or from being misused (not coming from your Heart). Not speaking up is a result of not trusting those around you or from not feeling safe enough to say what it is you have to say. Find other ways of expressing yourself to help open and strengthen your Throat chakra. Such things as singing to yourself or to your children, reading bedtime stories, or making up stories of your own to tell your children will help. Other effective tools are the use of mantras, chanting or toning a sound vibration. Mantras are the repetition of a phrase or sound, often said or sung to music. The mantra can have a personal or devotional meaning, or it can simply be a resonant syllable used to tune out external noises. Mantras work through sound to calm the mind. When chanted, the vibration of the sound helps to open the throat area. Toning is of the same nature, although it is simply repeating one resonant syllable to help open the throat. It does not matter what it is you do as long as you feel comfortable doing it, and as long as it involves using your voice and speaking out. Sound is key to opening the throat and it is the most effective tool you have to opening a closed Throat chakra. At the end of this chapter I have outlined the specific toning sounds associated with each chakra.

## Lessons from Chakra Five

### Communication

Sound, communication, and expressing ourselves is what the fifth chakra is all about. To commune with another is to merge with another. We learn that what we want to achieve in communication is to be heard, to be acknowledged, and to simply have a positive energy exchange. Defensive communication and the language you use sets up a block. As in your third chakra, try to avoid using judgmental or criticizing statements. The fifth chakra teaches you to strive for compassionate communication. Use "I" statements to bring you into your heart. If someone complains to you, ask them to take responsibility for themselves and use "I" statements, taking the "you" out of their statements.

## Think Before You Speak

From the fifth chakra we learn to be responsive rather than reactive. Reacting to a situation comes from generational learning. Holding or pausing when doing asanas teaches us to pause in life and in situations. We learn to think before we speak, and to come from the heart. We gain a perspective of the situation in order to see the bigger picture. We learn to trust and to let go, to have patience and tolerance. We learn to pause for a moment in order to make the right choice.

The fifth chakra has to do with your male energy, your more confident, outgoing, and assertive energy. Using this male energy helps you to learn to express with precision your thoughts and feelings about a situation rather than suppressing them. You learn to be brief, concise, and to the point. You learn to use the silence, the quiet moment, to connect and come from your heart; to express your thoughts without disempowering the next person. You learn to quiet your mind. Allow the gentle energy of the Heart chakra—love, compassion forgiveness—to enter your Throat chakra, blending with and softening the male energy of this chakra. Remember, you must go above the Throat chakra in order to heal it, to your Third Eye, which expresses a higher intuition.

## Speak Up

The fifth chakra teaches you to have the courage to feel fear and to express it. You learn to use quiet strength to express your fear, verbalizing it by coming from your Heart chakra. The Throat chakra gives you the power to speak the truth. This is the center where you may begin to feel fears in your own personal relationships—from not speaking up. We tend to pull back out of fear of not being loved. If you sense this happening in a relationship, admit there is a problem and start to change direction.

From the fifth chakra you learn to express the fine line and not use it as a control mechanism. Rather, you use it to empower both parties.

You learn to give others the freedom to express their needs, creating a safe environment for relationships to flourish. Aggression is having fear with the appearance of having no fear. It is lack of trust and the opposite of observing the fine line or using restraint.

## Toning Sounds for Each Chakra

As the specific syllable is toned for each chakra, its vibration resonates through your body, activating the energy within the corresponding chakra. Toning can be added to your daily yoga program as you go through the meditation of opening each chakra. The corresponding tones are as follows:[2]

| | |
|---|---|
| Chakra One | "O" as in "rope" |
| Chakra Two | "OO" as in "do" |
| Chakra Three | "OHM" |
| Chakra Four | "AY" as in "I" |
| Chakra Five | "AH" |
| Chakra Six | "EE" |
| Chakra Seven | "MM" |

The proper way to tone is to take in a deep breath through your nostrils, open your mouth, and sound the syllable as you exhale, continuing to sound until the last breath of air is used. This could take up to a minute, or longer, depending on the air capacity of your lungs. Repeat each syllable three times before moving on to the next one.

## Notes

1. Dr. Fedor Zelina, naturopath; Fazia Khan, certified yoga instructor, lecture notes, 1996–1997; Anodea Judith, *Wheels of Life: A User's Guide to the Chakra System* (Llewellyn Publications, 1987); Christiane Northrup, M.D., *Women's Bodies, Women's Wisdom* (Bantam Books, 1994).

2. Anodea Judith, *Wheels of Life: A User's Guide to the Chakra System* (Llewellyn Publications, 1987).

Chapter 26

# All About
# Chakra Six

*"I am intuitive."*

The sixth chakra, your Third Eye chakra and inner being, glows a deep indigo blue. It is located at the front part of your head in the center of your forehead, between and slightly above your eyebrows, with an opening at the back of the skull. The Third Eye relates to the activity and health of your mind.

The element associated with the sixth chakra is light, representing a flow of light and energy as you use your Third Eye to literally allow energy and knowledge to pour into you. Symbolically, light becomes knowledge as you use your Third Eye to "see" and "know" your inner knowledge. The Third Eye chakra is your source of creative energy and your ability to visualize. It is where you access the sort of knowledge you learn from listening to your internal feelings or hunches, the sort of knowledge that is beyond the reach of your senses. It is

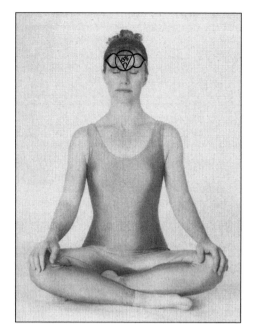

**Figure 26-1**

*The sixth chakra is your Third Eye chakra and inner being. It is located in the center of your forehead. It relates to the activity and health of your mind.*

your main source to the creative arts, where you access and receive intuition and inspiration through an open Third Eye. It is here that the designer visualizes her designs before drawing them, where the dancer feels the rhythm her dance before creating it, where the song artist hears his music before the notes are written.

The Third Eye chakra is associated with intellect, understanding, and clarity. It is here that you perceive higher concepts of the truth and begin to have an understanding of moral issues and the lessons you have to learn in your life. As your sixth chakra opens, your imagination and devotion increases. You have peace of mind but remain mentally very alert. Here too, it is important to remember to open the back of this chakra when opening the front. In order to implement the ideas that come to your Third Eye, your sixth chakra needs to be fully open. Opening the back of your this chakra clears your head of its congestion of thoughts, allowing your Third Eye to focus more clearly on the tasks at hand. Inner knowledge is accessed more easily and ideas processed through your Third Eye become more visible and intelligible to you. You can think more clearly and distinctly. When you have too much

## Chakra Six Table[1]

**Location:** The forehead, at the front of the head, behind the brow, and between the eyes

**Color:** Bright indigo blue

**Gland:** Pineal (gland of light)

**Organs:** The sixth chakra does not connect to any of the body's organs

**Body Parts:** Brain

**Function:**
Seeing
Intuition
Health of the mind
Healing (with wisdom and trust)

**Malfunction:**
Eye problems/blindness
Headaches, dizziness, Menieres disease
Parkinson's disease
Seizures
Brain tumors
Hemorrhages
Stroke
Learning disabilities, frustration
Nightmares
Misuse of intuition
Misuse of information (storytelling, deceit)

going on around you, it can be difficult to calm your mind sufficiently. Your head may feel like it has a build-up of pressure inside it, requiring an outlet to allow the pressure to ease. This is a common cause of headaches, or even migraines. If this happens, take a few minutes to relax your body and still your mind, using your breath. Imagine the discomfort leaving with your exhaling breath. Visualize a small hole opening at the back of your sixth chakra, and as you breathe, imagine the pressure and tension leaving through the opening, releasing the tension in the front of your head. I often get this feeling of pressure build-up when I try and tackle too many things in my day, not allowing myself to relax or enjoy myself. This visualization helps me a great deal, as well, it reminds me to slow down.

On a slightly different note, when you can not seem to get something out of your mind, play a mantra loudly in order to let the higher mind shift. As I explained in the previous chapter, a mantra is the repetition of a phrase or sound, often said to music. Mantras are very soothing to the mind and can work to "shift" it. You can not shift your mind through logic, that is, by asking it to stop thinking of whatever is stuck in your head. You can however, shift it with beauty.

A closed sixth chakra leads to someone being overly sensitive to the voice of reason, leading to an inflexible personality and someone not willing to take risks in life. Their life becomes dull and restricted. Hallucinating and overexaggerating stories are also signs of imbalance in this chakra.

The best way to strengthen and develop your sixth chakra is through meditation and visualization. When doing the Chakra Meditation, visualize the indigo blue color surrounding your head around the forehead area, both in the front and the back. Spend some time on this chakra as it can be a difficult one to open. Your Third Eye is located at the front of the head, behind your eyebrows and between your eyes. When in meditation, imagine your forehead opening up between your eyes. If you have a hard time visualizing this, simply ask it to open and know that it will. If you trust that it will open, the "feeling" that it is open will come. As you do this, visualize the back of the chakra opening as well, as mentioned earlier. Once the chakra is open fully, visualize the indigo blue light once again, as it wraps itself around your head. Try to feel the energy swirling around your head, and in and out through the openings in your sixth chakra. And now, spend some quiet time stilling your mind and asking for any inner knowledge that you need to know to come through at this time. The information will come. It may come in the form of pictures, music, or words, as in a thought. Do not expect flashes of information or do not look too hard, or you will miss it. Information comes to you gently and softly. It is easy to miss if you are not open to it. Once again, always acknowledge the information as it comes. And when something comes true as per your intuition, thank your intuition with gratitude for sending it to you. Acknowledge yourself and give yourself a pat on the back for being able to decipher it. You are beginning to trust your inner thoughts and perceptions. It is from here that you know that ideas can come true simply by putting them into action.

## Lessons From Chakra Six

### *Intuition*

As we learn to open our sixth chakra and learn to honor our intuitions and inspirations, the chakra grows in intensity and strength. Intuition has to do with trust, trusting the feeling of knowingness and that place from the heart, without fear of what may have happened in the past or what may happen in the future. It is about living in the present, in the moment. When you are able to trust being in the moment, and are comfortable with that, you are coming from your higher mind. Trusting yourself and living in the moment takes the stress out of living. It eases the flow of energy because you no longer feel divided by your past or future barriers. Living within an environment of trust, you open yourself to the ability of seeing new possibilities and other perspectives.

The Third Eye chakra is the place of your "inner knowing." You learn from this energy center that you can not walk the path of Oneness until you know how to walk the path of Wholeness. In other words, you need to claim your "self" back and get to know who you are. You can't be yourself until you know who you are.

It is through the sixth chakra that almost all the thoughts and messages you receive and send are interpreted. For this reason it is important that you learn to develop and strengthen the abilities of your Third Eye so that you recognize the fact that knowledge is coming through, and that this knowledge is often an opportunity for growth. As I write this book, I feel my sixth and seventh chakra open. I can feel knowledge coming through as it is channeled through my Crown and enters my Third Eye for processing. I feel this knowledge becoming a part of my being as I transfer my thoughts onto paper for you, the reader, to digest and benefit from as I do.

It is not only knowledge that comes through your sixth chakra, but it is here that your intuition is perceived, or felt. Intuition is an inner signal. As you open your heart and live from that place of being open, you are able to trust that feeling of "knowingness" and that place from the heart. You learn to trust your feelings of intuition as real, and as being safe. As you acknowledge and accept these feelings as real, your intuition becomes stronger. Intuition is a direct perception of truth or fact, independent from any reasoning process. The energy surrounding your being, your aura, is able to pick up on events happening around you because you are allowing yourself to "open up" to this energy. This is even true of events that will be happening in your future because the energy is out there coming your way. You are allowing yourself to be drawn to that energy so that you may be aware of it coming. If you learn to open up to this, you are able to decipher the knowledge as being useful and beneficial to your life. Your intuition is like your sixth sense, use it to your benefit. You are unique and special. When you ignore your feelings of intuition, the feelings begin to fade. Eventually, you will no longer be aware that they are even there.

## Breaking Patterns

Your sixth chakra can be disabled or impaired by the use of alcohol and/or drugs. It is in the this chakra that addictions or bad habits begin. But this is also the center where we are able to break away from old patterns. If you do not like a recurring pattern in your life (some-one hurting your feelings, money issues, worry, or any other pattern), then do not allow it to continue to be a part of your life. Break the pattern of allowing it to bother you. Release the negative feelings this pattern makes you feel. First, acknowledge the feeling. It is there to protect you and to let you know something is bothering you. Then, get in touch with that feeling and find out why this pattern bothers you. Why are your feelings hurt by what others say or do? Why are you worried about money? Allow yourself to release what bothers you and it will no longer be attracted to you. The process of breaking away from old patterns in order to reach your higher self is difficult. You need to have patience and be gentle on yourself. Your "old" self will probably kick and scream, fighting you along the way as you strive to change and find your way back to your higher path.

## Notes

1. Dr. Fedor Zelina, Naturopath; Fazia Khan, certified yoga instructor, lecture notes, 1996–1997; Anodea Judith, *Wheels of Life: A User's Guide to the Chakra System* (Llewellyn Publications, 1987); Christiane Northrup, M.D., *Women's Bodies, Women's Wisdom* (Bantam Books, 1994).

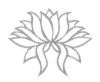

Chapter 27

# All About Chakra Seven

*"I am a being of pure light."*

The seventh chakra, your Crown chakra, is your higher self connection. Breathing through your Crown, centered at the top of your head, puts you in touch with your higher self, to God, and to spirit. The Crown chakra is shaped like a funnel at the top of your head, swirling with a violet purple light. As you work on opening your crown chakra, your external and internal lives are brought together, fusing together your body and spirit.

The element associated with the seventh chakra is thought, symbolizing eternity as it opens to achieve wisdom and spiritual union. It is through your Crown chakra that you are able to communicate with higher planes of consciousness and with your oneness with God. It is here that your Divine guidance is "known." When you take the time to call in the Divine, through

**Figure 23-1**

*The seventh chakra, your Crown chakra, is your higher self connection. Breathing through your Crown, centered at the top of your head, puts you in touch with your higher self, to God, and to spirit.*

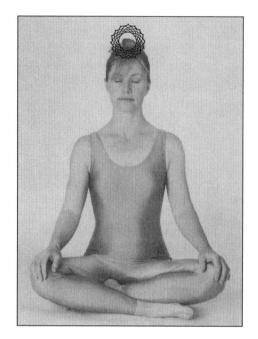

meditation, you realize you are a Divine Being. The Crown chakra is your God connection, and your connection to all things. You become aware of other planes of existence through your seventh chakra, and you have the courage to explore and examine them.

A balanced and open seventh chakra, along with the balancing of all the other chakras, is what we refer to as self-realization—understanding clearly who you are, who you have become, and acknowledging how you got there. As I explained previously, it is important to balance daily to maintain the balanced state of your chakras. You are continually growing and learning, and along the way you will come across barriers or obstructions that you need to learn how to overcome. Sometimes these barriers may seem like mountains that take awhile for us to climb and learn what it is we need to learn. Once we reach the top however, the lessons become clear, as does the way back to our path. Sometimes, if you are ready, a higher and more rewarding path is revealed. As you continue to grow, always remember your connection to your emotional body and the effect it has on your physical well-being. As you work to maintain a balanced and healthy chakra system,

## Chakra Seven Table[1]

| | |
|---|---|
| **Location:** | Top of the head |
| **Color:** | Violet purple |
| **Gland:** | Pituitary (master gland) |
| **Organs:** | The seventh chakra does not connect to any of the body's organs |
| **Function:** | Understanding<br>God connection |
| **Malfunction:** | Migraines<br>Depression, alienation<br>Inability to learn or comprehend<br>Developmental disorders<br>Genetic disorders<br>Multiple sclerosis<br>Confusion, boredom, apathy<br>Any life-threatening illness or accident serving as a wake-up call |

you agree to acknowledge challenge in your life, and you realize that if the difficulty is not attended to, it can begin to settle into your being, causing "dis-ease" on a physical level.

An open seventh chakra allows for a vivid imagination. You have a strong yet gentle personality and live your life unaffected by the personality traits that make you unique. An open seventh chakra leads to an acceptance of death without fear.

Working to open this chakra is easier than most people realize. When doing the Chakra Meditation, visualize an opening at the top of your head. If you can not visualize this, ask your Crown chakra to open, and it will. As in your seventh chakra, if you trust that the Crown chakra has opened, the "feeling" that it is opened will follow. Once you have experienced your seventh chakra as being opened, you won't want to turn back. As you learn to live your life with an open seventh chakra, you realize that living your life for materialistic reasons alone is no longer satisfying or sufficient. Your quest for a more spiritual connection has begun. This purple violet light of the seventh chakra is a purifying light, and as it enters your body through your Crown, allow its energy to heal you, purify you, and energize you.

With a closed seventh chakra, you will be unwilling or afraid to reach your spiritual potential and you will experience limited growth. You have a fear of death as well as a fear of enjoying life. It is here that you may develop a fear of God, the fear often stemming from a "victim consciousness" society or religion places on you. It has to do with your feelings of not being worthy. As you work to open your seventh chakra, you become aware of the sense that you are your own master. You choose your own thoughts. You are part of the light and co-create with your higher self and your connection to God. Take away the feelings of guilt you place on yourself. Realize that it is "you" placing these feelings on yourself, and no one else. You can continue to blame "others" for your problems, but it is not until you take responsibility for your own difficulty that you will be able to release the difficulty. It is "you" that is allowing these feelings to settle into your being and allowing them to become a part of who you are. If these feelings are not comfortable, then they are not serving your highest good. Release them when doing your chakra balancing. Find out where in your body you are feeling the discomfort. Go to that chakra and release the uncomfortable feelings before they become a block in your chakra. Once you do this you can enter the light and become one with your higher self and your connection to God.

## Lessons from Chakra Seven

### *Appreciate Life for the Right Reasons*

The seventh chakra teaches you how to live and become a part of your world without getting caught up in its misunderstandings and ignorance. It teaches you how to be a multidimensional being, as opposed to a three-dimensional being living in a three-dimensional, materialistic world. You are no longer impressed by people's external factors, as you are by what they are like on the inside. When studying yoga, my yoga instructor, Fazia, would say, "You are as the lotus flower, with its roots stuck in the mud but its flowers above the water, not getting caught up in the drama." What she meant was an open seventh chakra teaches us to keep our feet on the ground while looking up to the heavens for guidance. The lotus flower is the symbol used to depict the chakras, each petal of the flower symbolizing a specific physical and spiritual attribute. The Crown chakra is represented by a thousand petals, more than any of the other chakras.

### *Channel for Receiving Information and Knowledge*

You receive information and higher knowledge through your seventh chakra and when you do, you learn that you need to become hermit-like for awhile to allow the new knowledge to integrate with your body so that it feels comfortable, allowing the information to become a part of you. The function of being hermit-like is to allow you to replenish and get connected back to source, to fill up and be still. This is your chance to find your own personal path of abundance in life. You learn to be self-sufficient and self-reliant and you learn to love yourself. Taking the time to reflect within allows you to see and recognize your "fear" patterns that prevent you from moving forward.

It is at your Crown chakra that your masters and guides come down to meet you. We have masters and guides that are always with us. With them, they carry knowledge that is specific to your well-being, and this knowledge is available and accessible to you at any time. You just need to ask for it. These beings vibrate at a higher energy than you do, and if you want to meet them, you need to go up to their energy level. They are unable to come down to yours. When working with spirit guides it is important that you remain clear and receptive in your sixth chakra, your Third Eye, as it is here that you receive their messages. It is their messages that we often receive in the form of intuition or perception. When you are open to their energy, you can feel their presence, and will immediately have a sense as to who they are. If you wish to work with spirit guides to enhance and accelerate you spiritual growth, you can ask for their guidance at any time, and are encouraged to use the abilities of your Third Eye to receive their messages.

## Notes

1. Dr. Fedor Zelina, naturopath; Fazia Khan, certified yoga instructor, lecture notes, 1996–1997; Anodea Judith, *Wheels of Life: A User's Guide to the Chakra System* (Llewellyn Publications, 1987); Christiane Northrup, M.D., *Women's Bodies, Women's Wisdom* (Bantam Books, 1994).

# Bibliography

Ansari, Mark and Liz Lark. *Yoga for Beginners*. Harper Collins, 1998.

Feurstein, George. *The Shambhala Encyclopedia*. Shambhala Publications, Inc., 1997.

Hay, Louise L. *You Can Heal Your Life*. Hay House, 1994.

Judith, Anodea. *The Wheels of Life: A Study Guide for the Chakras*. Llewellyn Publications, 1987.

Khan, Fazia. Yoga classes/lecture notes. Center of the Emerald Heart Natural Healing Services, Richmond Hill, Ontario, 1996–97.

Northrup, Christiane. *Women's Bodies, Women's Wisdom*. Bantam Books, 1994.

Ohlendorf-Moffat, Pat. "Body & Soul Chakra Meditation." *Pathways*. September/October, 1993.

Peck, Scott M. *The Road Less Traveled*. Simon and Schuster, Inc., 1978.

Roseborough, Kathie. Meditation classes/lecture notes. Aurora Healing Arts Center, 1994–96.

Winter Ward, Susan. "Yoga for the Young at Heart." *The Natural Way*. November/December, 1996.

Zebroff, Kareen. *ABC of Yoga.* Forbez Publications, Limited,1997.

Zelina, Dr. Fedor. Class notes/handouts on spinal contacts of the chakras. Center of the Emerald Heart Natural Healing Services, Richmond Hill, Ontario, 1996.

# Index

# ☾ REACH FOR THE MOON

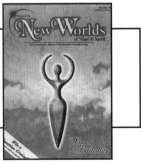

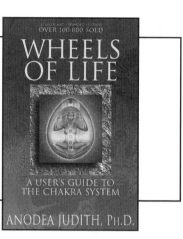

## Wheels of Life
### *A User's Guide to the Chakra System*

### ANODEA JUDITH, PH.D.

*Wheels of Life* is an instruction manual for owning and operating the inner gears that run the machinery of our lives. Written in a practical, down-to-earth style, this fully illustrated book will take the reader on a journey through aspects of consciousness, from the bodily instincts of survival to the processing of deep thoughts.

Discover this ancient metaphysical system under the new light of popular Western metaphors: quantum physics, Kabbalah, physical exercises, poetic meditations, and visionary art. Learn how to open these centers in yourself, and see how the chakras shed light on the present world crises we face today. And learn what you can do about it!

This book will be a vital resource for: magicians, witches, pagans, mystics, yoga practitioners, martial arts people, psychologists, medical people, and all those who are concerned with holistic growth techniques.

The modern picture of the chakras was introduced to the West largely in the context of hatha and Kundalini yoga and through the Theosophical writings of Leadbeater and Besant. But the chakra system is equally innate to Western Magick: all psychic development, spiritual growth, and practical attainment is fully dependent upon the opening of the chakras!

**0-87542-320-5, 528 pp., 6 x 9, illus.**                               **$17.95**

### To order, call 1-800-THE MOON
Prices subject to change without notice